Folk Healing and Health Care Practices in Britain and Ireland

Series: Epistemologies of Healing

General Editors: David Parkin, Fellow of All Souls College, University of Oxford, and Elisabeth Hsu, ISCA, University of Oxford

This series in medical anthropology will publish monographs and collected essays on indigenous (so-called traditional) medical knowledge and practice, alternative and complementary medicine, and ethnobiological studies that relate to health and illness. The emphasis of the series is on the way indigenous epistemologies inform healing, against a background of comparison with other practices, and in recognition of the fluidity between them.

Volume 1
Conjuring Hope: Magic and Healing in Contemporary Russia
Galina Lindquist

Volume 2
Precious Pills: Medicine and Social Change among Tibetan Refugees in India
Audrey Prost

Volume 3
Working with Spirit: Experiencing Izangoma Healing in Contemporary South Africa
Jo Thobeka Wreford

Volume 4
Dances with Spiders: Crisis, Celebrity and Celebration in Southern Italy
Karen Lüdtke

Volume 5
'The Land Is Dying': Contingency, Creativity and Conflict in Western Kenya
Paul Wenzel Geissler and Ruth J. Prince

Volume 6
Plants, Health and Healing: On the Interface of Ethnobotany and Medical Anthropology
Edited by Elisabeth Hsu and Stephen Harris

Volume 7
Morality, Hope and Grief: Anthropologies of AIDS in Africa
Edited by Hansjörg Dilger and Ute Luig

Volume 8
Folk Healing and Health Care Practices in Britain and Ireland: Stethoscopes, Wands and Crystals
Edited by Ronnie Moore and Stuart McClean

Folk Healing and Health Care Practices in Britain and Ireland

Stethoscopes, Wands and Crystals

Edited by

Ronnie Moore and Stuart McClean

Berghahn Books
New York • Oxford

First published in 2010 by

Berghahn Books

www.berghahnbooks.com

Library of Congress Cataloging-in-Publication Data

Folk healing and health care practices in Britain and Ireland : stethoscopes, wands, and crystals / edited by Ronnie Moore and Stuart McClean.

p. cm. -- (Epistemologies of healing)

Includes bibliographical references and index.

ISBN 978-1-84545-672-6 (hardback : alk. paper)

1. Traditional medicine--Great Britain--Formulae, receipts, prescriptions. 2. Traditional medicine--Ireland--Formulae, receipts, prescriptions. 3. Alternative medicine--Great Britain. 4. Alternative medicine--Ireland. 5. Healing--Great Britain. 6. Healing--Ireland. I. Moore, Ronnie. II. McClean, Stuart.

GR141.F59 2010

610.941--dc22

2010018158

British Library Cataloguing in Publication Data

A catalogue record for this book is available from the British Library

Printed in the United States on acid-free paper

ISBN 978-1-84545-672-6 (hardback)

Contents

For Rebecca Sarah and Lucy Constance

Acknowledgements

There are many people we would like to thank. Firstly, thanks to all of the contributors who shared their research. We would like to thank the generosity of Dr Andrew Sanders and Professor Michael Laffan for reading early drafts of the chapters and for giving advice and encouragement. In addition, we thank the external reviewers. None of the above share any responsibility for any errors, factual or otherwise. Catherine Cox's research was supported by the Wellcome Trust. Thanks also go to Dr Sibylle Naglis. Anne MacFarlane and Tomas de Brún gratefully acknowledge the enormous contribution of the CARe peer researchers. Also the contributions made by the Health Services Executive, Western Area (Departments of Health Promotion and Primary Care) and the Galway Refugee Support Group. Thanks also go to Mary O'Reilly de Brún and Helen Lambert for their comments.

We would like to say thanks to our friends and colleagues who sustain us through difficult times. We thank also Northern Ireland Railway and the staff of the (Belfast–Dublin) Enterprise train, where much of this book was drafted and revised. Finally, thanks to our families in Belfast and Bristol who have supported us and put up with our occasional absences.

Ronnie and Stuart.

Chapter 1

Introduction: Folk Healing in Contemporary Britain and Ireland: Revival, Revitalisation or Reinvention?

Ronnie Moore and Stuart McClean

Christ and Rasputin number among the many folk healers in history. The practice is both ubiquitous and unique. It is at once a familiar and shared socio-cultural phenomenon, but it also evokes something magical and other, distant and irrational, and it is seen as deeply antithetical to 'modern' ways of thinking and being. And therein we can locate the complexity of addressing a subject both familiar and alien in a modern society which is assumed to be in the process of shedding the 'last vestiges' of such non-scientific and premodern beliefs and practices.

In sharing the topic of this book with colleagues, we have noted that a similar theme emerges, in which the mention of 'folk cures' brings to light other people's sometimes remarkable experiences and memories of relatives and extended kin who have been 'blessed' with the ability to cure or, at least, to offer solace and comfort to those in need. Unlike the many and varied complementary and alternative health practitioners in Britain and Ireland, folk healers are not easily discovered, and it is this undefined, unrefined and incomplete picture that we have of folk healing practices in these regions that further complicates, but also enriches, our narrative.

Many of us, and not just the contributors to this book, have witnessed a folk cure, or have overheard a story revealing a folk wisdom, although more than likely it was not seen as a 'folk' act at the time. More commonly held beliefs that derive from folk conceptualisations – 'an apple a day', 'feed a cold, starve a fever', eating a hot breakfast on a cold day – are not necessarily perceived as folk wisdom as they have entered mainstream, sometimes even biomedical, consciousness and have thus become 'common sense'.

There are uneasy aspects of this in folk healing, as it has often been perceived as denoting health beliefs that are erroneous – magical superstitions, or 'old wives' tales', with their own set of assumptions of gendered knowledge (Hufford 1997). This is problematic in the main, as modern medicine has appropriated aspects of folk knowledge in its practice. Also, the relationship between folk medicine and biomedicine has often been seen as two-way (Helman 1986). Thus, far from contesting the lay or folk view of colds and fevers, the biomedical germ theory of disease, Helman suggests, actually supports it. The boundaries of knowledge between the folk and the medical (and expert) are, at least within areas of anthropological inquiry, perceived as fluid and contestable.

Indeed, in this book we highlight the interdependent and interactional nature of biomedical, folk and other alternative and complementary treatments. The boundaries between heterodox folk and complementary and alternative medicine (CAM) practices, as well as biomedicine, are perceived as both contestable and fluid. It will become clear that the various competing healing practices, ideologies and healthcare fields collude with and challenge each other (and have done so historically), and therefore the book will be of relevance to those interested in biomedicine as well as folk, alternative and complementary medicine.

Folk healing is not just about 'tradition', and within an anthropological framework we need to be careful about 'exoticising' such practices, or of over-emphasising their significance in a British and Irish healthcare context. The sentiment in this volume is that folk healing is not about the 'few surviving vestiges of premodern medical thought' (Hufford 1992: 15); folk healing can be 'modern', contemporary, rooted in everyday life and communities, and it is concerned with the here and now. And yet it is also the other side to modernity, it represents a challenge to and a competing (and necessary) alternative discourse to Western science.

One of the uniting themes in this book, then, is to provide illustrative, ethnographic and anthropological examples of folk-healing knowledge and practices, as well as those practices on the boundaries of what is deemed 'folk', and to consider what picture they present about folk healing and healthcare in Britain and Ireland at the beginning of the twenty-first century. In presenting these empirical cases we suggest that in order to answer adequately the question 'what is folk medicine?' one must explore the phenomenon in the context in which it emerges and is practised. This must, above all, be an argument situated in embedded knowledge, for folk-healing knowledge too is 'situated knowledge' (Napolitano and Flores 2003).

This book begins by locating the rise of biomedical culture in the modern period. It discusses the eclipse and subsequent rediscovery and influence of folk medicine and addresses the expansion and changing legitimacy of alternative and complementary medicine in the postmodern era. It begins by introducing health concepts, beliefs and healthcare practices in the early modern period and considers their continuing relevance. Uniquely, it brings together in discussion recent interdisciplinary, cross-cultural examples of folk healing and informal healthcare practices within Britain and Ireland. The diversity of comparative ethnographic field studies adds considerable weight to the broader theoretical discussion of folk medicine.

Definitional Parameters: Warts 'n' All

Unashamedly interdisciplinary in nature, folk medicine has been the object of study for a range of academic disciplines, including social and cultural anthropology, folklore studies, history, ethnology, ethnopharmacology, ethnobotany and sociology, and more lately, public-health medicine. Folk medicine has inevitably been seen as being tied to particular subcultural groups, such as ethnic subgroups, reinforcing the notion of the 'popular stereotype of folk medicine as marginal to modern culture' (Hufford 1988: 243). Equally and inevitably, this stereotype is also reinforced by much of the medical literature.[1]

Previous texts giving space exclusively to addressing folk medicine have sometimes taken an encyclopaedic approach to documenting the range of folk practices and cures cross-culturally, and in this endeavour an enormous variety of magical folk cures have been documented in the U.S., Europe and elsewhere (see Hand 1980). Further, there is a large body of writing on the efficacy of folk 'pharmacology' and the knowledge of healing properties of medicinal plants and plant roots (Hand 1980; Croom 1992; Mathews 1992), trees (Levine 1941; Earwood 1999), and other natural substances used as curative agents (see Wahlberg, this volume).

Much of the writing on complementary and alternative medicine (increasingly known as the acronym CAM), for example, makes little or no mention of folk medicine or folk healing, as noted previously by Hufford (1997). Where it is given some attention it has been in relation to the general approach to various forms of unorthodoxy highlighting its commonality with non-orthodox drugs and interventions, religious healing, and health crusades (Gevitz 1988). Here the emphasis is on the absence of organising motifs and themes that would allow one to make a useful comparison between such a broad range of practices. Thus, unorthodox practitioners are a 'heterogeneous population promoting disparate beliefs and practices which vary considerably from one movement to another and form no consistent or complementary body of knowledge' (ibid.: 1).

A central dilemma in unpacking the influence and continuing effect of folk-health practices is their scope. The majority of studies of folk-healing practices and beliefs, perhaps understandably, have focused on pre-industrial societies rather than on industrial and post-industrial ones. Undeniably the literature is extensive and others have produced voluminous accounts of folk healing practices, from the regional ethnically linked traditions of *curanderismo* in Mexico and the south-western U.S.A. (Trotter and Chavira 1997), to the *espiritismo* of Hispanic Puerto Ricans, and the 'burn' healers of eastern North Carolina (Kirkland 1992), but that is not the aim of this book. Clearly folk healing and health practices are inevitably tied up with, and sometimes hardly indistinguishable from, regional and local ethnic 'traditions'; the heterogeneity of the population will undoubtedly affect the diversity of the folk 'tradition' (Hufford 1988). Indeed, as Hufford states, anthropological definitions of folk medicine generally see the folk as located between the local, indigenous traditions and the 'official' or 'informal' medical system of the 'culture'; 'unofficial' or 'informal' therefore designates a useful starting point for any debate about folk healing.

Folk, moreover, has often been used generically to refer to all those practices that 'lie outside the "normal" sphere of operations of orthodox Western medical practice' (Bakx 1991: 21). This is a useful definition, although we are likely to narrow this down slightly, since this would provide too broad a range of health practices, in addition to providing semantic as well as epistemological difficulties over what constitutes a 'normal sphere of operations'. In Bakx's definition the practices of complementary and alternative medicine (CAM) are included, and although we would question their incorporation into a 'folk' model, there are useful questions raised here about the folk-inspired nature of many so-called alternative therapies (see McClean, this volume).

Included in these broad definitions, therefore, would be other practices such as the use of 'natural' folk remedies and folk herbalism (see Wahlberg, this volume), in addition to natural health foods and the health movement more generally, originating in the U.S. in the 1950s (Hufford 1988). Further, it is possible in constructing a text on folk health and healing practices that we have also to open ourselves to a discussion of folk illness and other localised socio-medical phenomena (culture-bound syndromes), so intertwined are the concepts.

There is however a wider debate about the extent to which the same concept can be used to analyse such a diverse range of different observable phenomena. As Alver explains, 'The folk system is indeed heterogeneous; there may be greater differences than similarities between the various treatment categories' (Alver 1995: 24). One of the aims of this volume, then, is to provide greater clarity over the scope of folk healing and its relationship both to Western scientific medicine and other alternative health modalities.

Suffice to say, in this book we retain a more fluid, flexible and contextual model and definition of folk medicine, in which the knowledge, discourses and practices of various healing modalities interact and intersect at both pragmatic and symbolic levels. What is useful at this stage is to consider some of the debates so far, to begin to construct a typology of folk healing, and to unpick what might constitute the ideal type. In the following we briefly refer to the issues raised in the literature and select some common themes. Further, we highlight, where necessary, the links between the features of folk healing and the chapters in this volume.

Towards a Classification of Folk Healing

Because it is a contested field there is obvious disagreement amongst writers as to what constitutes folk healing or, the more ubiquitous phrase in the literature, folk medicine. In this book we maintain a preference for the term folk healing (although we utilise both as appropriate), with connotations less of the interventionist and curing aspects of the medical model, and more of the supplementary, caring aspects of the lay model. However, what is clear is that authors are in broad agreement about the particular features of what might constitute folk healing, and we expand on some of these themes below.

Writers on folk healing and medicine have pulled together the various features that gives them their distinctive character and have highlighted their difference from Western scientific biomedicine and other forms of complementary and alternative medicine. A number of these features are too similar to other CAM: 'nature', wholeness and purity (Vaskilampi 1981). To our mind, folk medicine is not indistinguishable from CAM therapies, but we need to underline an important distinction here.

Hufford (1988, 1997) highlights the importance of the predominance of the transmission of oral knowledge, although he notes that few healing beliefs could exist completely independent of other media. Other common elements include a reliance on such terms as 'energy' (Hufford 1988, 1997), where folk traditions are closely linked to the concept of vitalism. Here the debate concerns the nature of folk healing as the transfer of 'good' energies into the patients in order to deal with the negative energies absorbed by the patient or client.

Folk Healing as Informal Lay Medicine

Folk healing is relatively informal in structure, when compared to the more institutionalised scientific biomedicine. We have focused on folk practices' emphasis on the informal nature of the learning process and form of knowledge transmission, in which particular folk techniques and embodied practice are transmitted by significant others, family and friends. In line with Kleinman's (1980) general model of healthcare sectors, where the folk, popular and professional sectors interact, we can see how folk healing retains its power and influence surrounding everyday healthcare decisions. Folk healing in this sense is practised by lay people who are not legally recognised as professionals (see Stone, this volume) and do not enjoy a protected status (De Wert 1984). And yet, 'In the eyes of the local people they are, however, acknowledged specialists' (ibid.: 104). In a pluralistic health culture there is likely to be a degree of tension and conflict between these different competing sectors. 'Folk wisdom' may be more significant than visiting the doctor, and the role of informal networks in aiding that process is crucially important.

It is the informal nature of such folk healing practices that lead some to see these characteristics as promoting a different type of expertise and authority, one that is not based on the formal aspects accorded to professional expert-based knowledge systems. As 'unofficial' knowledge, folk healing lacks authority structures, but is able to compensate for this in ways more meaningful to those who utilise it: 'Folk medicine carries authority, but it is the informal authority of life experience rather than the formal authority of licensure, certification and accreditation' (Hufford 1997: 726).

Thus, folk practices, in tandem with 'traditional' ones, are often perceived as being informally led and based on a less institutionalised form of knowledge transmission. Kirkland et al. point out that the term 'folk' is used 'to designate any medical concept or behaviour based on non-institutionalised oral traditional practices rather than on formal academic and clinical training' (Kirkland et al. 1992: ix). The process of informal learning means that the learning of specific healing practices may come from friends and family, originating perhaps in childhood (Croom 1992), or from other healers who sense the healing potential in others.

In considering the informal (and potentially 'disorganised') aspects of folk healing, others have focused on the ways in which folk-healing practices are symbolic of deeper, more culturally embedded 'lay' practices and therefore should not be analysed separately from other lay phenomena. Here folk healing is a 'deeply embedded, unorganized, and seemingly spontaneous response to illness ... confined to specific geographical areas ... magical traditions or earlier lay forms of self-care and home remedies' (Kaptchuk and Eisenberg 2001: 200). Undoubtedly folk healing practices do not require similar levels of organisation and systematised knowledge as more 'global', scientific systems of knowledge such as Western biomedicine. Its 'informal' nature, with its roots in lay knowledge, are also its strengths as a form of healing knowledge that is more in sympathy with the localities and communities it treats.

Folk healing is considered to include practices that involve a degree of apprenticeship (Hänninen 1981; Hufford 1997), and, although the transmission of knowledge from one person to another is not in doubt, the extent of this apprenticeship is, as is its relative significance across a range of culturally specific folk-medical forms. Here the emphasis is on folk healing as a craft, where particular skills are handed down through successive generations, Evans-Pritchard's description of the transmission of medical (magical) knowledge amongst the Azande being the 'classic' anthropological example:

> Men who possess medicines of a specialized activity, like witch-doctors and those who practise the blacksmith's art, pass on their knowledge to one of their sons when he learns the craft. Likewise, a man who knows valuable medicine, like vengeance-magic, teaches it bit by bit to a favourite son over a long period of time, for several rare plants and other objects often furnish different elements in the magical compound. Old men sometimes hand over a treasured charm, like the whistle which gives invisibility, to a son as an heirloom. (Evans-Pritchard 1976: 186)

Folk Healing as Gift versus the 'Calling'

In this book there are examples of how those who practice folk healing refer to their involvement in healing as a 'calling' (Alver 1981; McClean, this volume), or alternatively those who were born into it (see Lee-Treweek, this volume). This debate mirrors that highlighted by MacCormack (1981) concerning the difference between ascribed healers (those who claim healing as a birth right) and healers by achievement (where others recognise the individual's healing ability). There are subtle differences between the two: whereas a 'calling' suggests the process of apprenticeship occurring after the 'revelatory moment', being born into it denotes the healer's power as their birth right (see also Philpin, this volume).

For those that are 'called' to heal there are questions about the status of the latter kind of healers and their wider role within the community. The idea of the 'calling' is often that the healer does not have the ability to heal but is a conduit for healing 'energies'; they are a channel for other, more benign, spiritual powers. One of the most prominent specialists in the area of folklore and folk medicine, Wayland Hand (1971), explored how the 'gift' of folk healing is acquired by an individual in three distinct ways: a gift specially conferred; a gift innate in the healer; and a gift resulting from a unique condition. For Hand, the gift is often linked to the date and time of birth, position in the lineage, or a person's name. A central theme in his work has been to highlight the importance of birth right in conferring the status of folk healer:

> By the very fact that such healers are specially marked and derive their power and virtue as healers from the accidents of birth and station, it is clear that the usual means of perpetuating the gift are totally unavailing … Nor does one hear of the conferral of the healer's gift from one sex to another, or any kind of transmission, personal or otherwise. (ibid.: 274–75)

Between Individuation and Systematisation: Folk Healing as 'Modern' Cultural Practice

There is some level of debate, not just in relation to folk healing but across the full range of alternative health practices, about the tension between the need for individuals to express their own forms of healing practice and the importance of key principles and rules of practice, however loosely defined. This tension is often theorised as a difference between individuation and systematisation (see McClean 2003, 2005), or individuation and depersonalisation (Broom and Tovey 2007).

In focusing on individuation, such writers have explored both the creative and potentially empowering aspect of these practices, as well as the 'darker' side, where ideologies of blame and individual responsibility may also predominate (McClean 2005). Other writers on folk healing have also focused on the strong moral undertones of such practices, where exposing oneself to illness may be seen as an imbalance resulting from individuals neglecting to protect themselves adequately. There is 'common reference to personal responsibility in folk medicine' (Hufford 1997: 726). In these examples, illness is the result of personal misfortune, viewed and treated the same way as divorce, losing a job or the break-up of a relationship (Snow 1978).

The literature on folk medicine and folk healing displays some uncertainty about the extent to which these practices constitute 'systems', as opposed to being seen as just another illustration of 'cultural flotsam and jetsam' (Hufford 1997: 736). In her discussion of folk practices in the eastern regions of North Carolina and Virginia, for example, Mathews (1992) refers to the practices as 'systems'. Hufford likewise accords folk medicine the status of 'system', constituted in a similar, but not altogether identical, way to biomedicine: 'folk medicine [consists of] systems that interact with the other systems of belief present within North American culture (including the beliefs of modern medicine)' (Hufford 1988: 253).

The folk sector has been characterised as an 'open' system, in that it interacts freely with other social institutions: the family, the economic sector, rituals, and so on (Press 1978). Alver (1981) talks of folk medicine as an open system that responds to need as it arises, embedded as it is within the community, whereas biomedicine is a closed system, global rather than local, and one that is locked into a priori assumptions. It is a closed system as it is based on precisely defined ('universal') knowledge and procedures that are not contextual: it does not depend on place and time, or practitioner (Press 1978).

A theme developed in this volume is that folk practices (because they are an open system) are more likely to serve the psychosocial needs of the community they are located in. This is in contrast to scientific medicine, where communities experience a lack of control and power over external threats, or events they perceive as beyond their sphere of influence (Snow 1978; Mathews 1987, 1992): 'health problems are inextricably linked with other matters of daily life, lack of money, loss of a job, envious neighbors, a straying spouse' (Snow 1978: 102). As Press explains, 'An *open* system is an *adaptive* system' (Press 1978: 72): it adapts to new social and environmental changes and threats. Press highlights how folk medicine, as the material and symbolic expression of specific cultural forms, can help migrants adapt to new urban environments.

In relation to Black American folk healers, such as root doctors (variously referred to in the literature as voodoo, hoodoo, witchcraft and hexing), this social theme concerning the use of folk medicine to address the lack of control individuals have over their lives has been particularly central; it continues to apply to the more economically deprived Black and minority, ethnic communities and areas in the U.S. Many Black and minority ethnic groups in the U.S. are perceived as alienated from orthodox medicine, and when it is used it is often in tandem with folk treatments (Scott 1974). Here racism, and the extent of social inequality, social uncertainty and poverty amongst Black American communities, can reveal more about the nature of folk healing and the extent and meanings behind its everyday usage.

The Scope and Outline of the Book

This volume is divided into three parts. Part I considers the historical context of folk healing (Introduction and Chapter 2 and 3). It introduces the history of healing practices, health beliefs and healthcare. These chapters examine the rise of biomedicine and draw upon varied contemporary and theoretical accounts of folk medicine. The late eighteenth and nineteenth centuries saw the broadening of access to 'formal' medical provision. This took the form of the emergence of regular practitioners, the expansion of institutional provision and, in the late nineteenth century, the professionalisation of medicine. It has often been assumed that this process led to the displacement of older existing practices of medical healing.

In Chapter 2, Moore and McClean outline how biomedicine has acquired a privileged place as a healthcare practice in Western society. Its hegemonic position is cemented through science's association with authoritative expert knowledge. Biomedicine has acted as a gatekeeper over the label 'science', which in turn helps defend its interests and achieve professional closure. However, while folk healing has not undergone a formally recognised process of rehabilitation, the continuance or re-emergence of alternative health practices underscores a major socio-cultural transformation, one in which 'expertise' is challenged and personalised knowledge celebrated. We can refer to this era as post-scientific, although a range of explanations are explored. Science is the most culturally embedded and reflexive system of knowledge in Western society, so changes to the status of science have fundamental implications for the nature and legitimacy of knowledge in a post-scientific era. This chapter locates the emergence of biomedicine's dominance in the context of modernity. It examines the rise and professionalism of biomedicine and draws upon varied contemporary and theoretical accounts of folk medicine. The professional nature of scientific knowledge, the increasing professionalisation of complementary and alternative medicine (CAM), and the changing nature of legitimacy are discussed in relation to the emerging social context. The chapter also considers the role and meaning of informal healing practices in a post-scientific era, where science and forms of expert knowledge are questioned. It concludes with a summary of the challenges folk healing poses to scientific knowledge in more local contexts.

The chapter further elaborates on the historical aspects of folk healing, locating this within wider sociological and anthropological debates. In so doing, it brings to bear a number of theoretical positions and discusses folk healing in a modern, late modern or postmodern context. It deals with cosmology; ancient as well as contemporary cross cultural interpretations of health and illness; traditional health beliefs and 'survivals' of formerly mainstream beliefs; and how these have been reframed and reinterpreted in the wake of dominant (and imported) religious beliefs. It also discusses the juxtaposition (and we would contend, false paradox) of science and religion and the intimate relationship between faith and medicine. The paradigmatic schisms produced by the Enlightenment and concomitant spiritual, social, economic, cultural and cognitive changes are also discussed. So too is the emergence and development of modern (or formal) medicine, and science as the direction of, and justificatory rhetoric for, biological medicine. It also addresses the elitist and protectionist practice of formal medicine (now with global tendencies).

Drawing on the National Folklore Collection, and archives at University College Dublin, in Chapter 3 Cox explores the historical literature, looking at the relationship between folk medicine, local health beliefs and regular and irregular medical practice in Ireland. She also explores the factors influencing the acceptance of practitioners 'regular and informal' by communities, and assesses the importance of economics, reputation and 'ethical' behaviour upon the practitioner's chances of success or failure. In so doing, Cox draws out the tensions between traditional and formal healthcare practices, pointing up lay pragmatism based on perceived efficacy, culturally preferred treatments and costs.

Part II presents a wide range of contemporary, ethnographically informed, research into 'indigenous' health practices. In Chapter 4, Philpin introduces wool measuring as a particular type of folk healing, described in Welsh folk literature from the late nineteenth and early twentieth centuries, that has survived in parts of rural mid Wales to the present day. The most common form of illness for which wool measuring is currently sought is the condition that people define as 'depression' (*clefyd-y-galon*). As Philpin observes, the act of wool measuring was symbolic of ethnic belonging, with responsibilities such as acceptance of certain codified behaviour and adhering to an indigenous, localised belief system and knowledge. The study emphasises the relationship between the individual and the community, and how ill health was mediated by community processes via the folk healer through the process of wool measuring. It emphasises an essentially Durkheimian quality, that of the primacy of the will of the group over the individual and importantly how this translates into therapy and efficacy for sufferers of depression. Philpin (like Moore in Chapter 5) highlights the relationship between folk healing and local economics in the form of animal husbandry. She argues that people turn to traditional medicine where biomedicine is unsuccessful, because the conditions do not fit easily into biomedical classifications.

In Chapter 5, Moore outlines findings from ethnographic research which set out to look at health and the assessment of related need in two small rural towns (one Catholic and one Protestant) in Northern Ireland. The research was conducted in an area variously described as 'the murder triangle' and 'bandit country'. Moore presents hitherto unreported information on the crucial role that folk healing played in the lives of people in these communities. He focuses on beliefs and ideas about health (both lay and professional), and the role of informal or folk healing in these communities and how they were integrated into general healthcare practice in both communities. Moore discusses the practice of folk healing known locally as 'the cure' or 'charm', and the centrality of this for local belief systems: how it impacted on the social and economic structure of both communities, and how this was seen to operate – that is, how and by what mechanisms 'the cure' or 'charm' was inherited or transferred. It also highlights the interface between local people and formal health care systems, the role of folk medicine and the bridge between folk medicine and modern medicine.

The first community studied was the Catholic town of Ballymacross and initial analysis suggested that belief in the 'cure/charm' was more likely to be tied to a specifically Catholic ethos (defined in an ethnic, cultural and religious sense). Only after fieldwork was carried out in Protestant Hunterstown did the full extent of the embeddedness of 'cures/charms' become known, transcending religious affiliation in these polarised communities. A central point made by Moore is that folk healing is not, (*pace* some of the literature), confined to Catholics and Catholicism, but is alive and well in Protestant communities in Northern Ireland.

Herbal medicine is seen as a part of folk medicine, albeit a separate part with a scientific edge. In Chapter 6, Wahlberg investigates the demise, revival and resurgent interest in British herbal medicine. He shows how the British medical establishment, by legally challenging indigenous herbal practices, drove them to the brink of extinction. Wahlberg makes the link between local folk medicine and folk medicine from other countries and healthcare systems, including Ayurvedic, Tibetan and Chinese medicine. He shows that practitioners of British herbal medicine now incorporate aspects of imported Asian and Latin American medicine into their repertoire of healing plants.

He also emphasises the belief that it is the failure of biomedicine (as people have become alienated from a formalised, depersonalised and bureaucratic system) that has revived folk medical traditions. Wahlberg discusses the value of twentieth-century anthropology to understanding the emic worldviews of peoples and underscores the need to document and go 'back to the roots' of herbal medicine to rescue original country (appropriate) remedies and folk recipes that have been used for centuries. As with MacFarlane and de Brún (Chapter 8, this volume), he also underscores how globalising forces and traditions from other healthcare systems are influencing and shaping healthcare and medical knowledge in Britain. He argues that indigenous herbal medicine in Britain has reinvented itself as Western herbal medicine, as distinct from its Chinese, Ayervedic or Tibetan variants.

In Chapter 7, McClean introduces ethnographic research on alternative health practices in the form of crystal and spiritual healing. Spiritual healing has its roots in the spiritualist practices of nineteenth-century Victorian society. However, he not only considers the resurgence of such practices but also introduces a discussion of features that are new to the contemporary scene. He discusses how crystal healing and spiritual healing are commonly practised at centres that exert little regulatory control. McClean focuses on one such centre in Northern England that is organised and run by a charismatic and entrepreneurial healer. While the practice is personalised, healing is sanctioned by the Centre and by the leader of the Centre. This situation can be seen as particularly paradoxical, and McClean offers a range of illustrative examples.

Within his discussion he unearths the importance of the 'trance' and communication between the living and the dead. While the spiritual sceptics remained unconvinced of this form of communication – in the famous case of the escapologist Harry Houdini, it was not disbelief per se, but the inability of a grieving son to contact his deceased mother – other notables, such as the physician Sir Arthur Conan Doyle, were persuaded. The chapter considers the resurgence and revitalisation of folk-inspired spiritual practices. Crystal healing has been bracketed as one of a number of neo-pagan and New Age treatments when in fact, as McClean shows, its roots stem from a much earlier time. This is an eclectic mix of New Age reference to Christ with aspects of seemingly more pagan beliefs and rituals in the use of crystals and symbolic trappings, including paraphernalia and metaphors of biomedicine.

McClean shows that crystal and spiritual healing, unlike other forms of folk healing, are representative of a seemingly more organised and centralised (and quasi-professional) practice, even though the actual practice of healing is personalised. This rests on institutional philosophy and peer approval and diverges from other traditional folk-healing practices that emphasise the non-centralised, indigenous, local and informal. He makes links between crystal and spiritual healing and CAM. The examples used are illustrative of the disillusionment experienced by patients who perceive formal medical care as having given up on them.

In Chapter 8, MacFarlane and de Brún approach health issues of migrants in the wake of what has came to be called 'the Celtic tiger'; that is, the unprecedented patterns of migration into the Republic of Ireland as a result of its recent economic success (though this may now be more accurately described as a 'paper tiger'). They look at plural health practices of Serbo-Croat and Russian-speaking refugees and asylum seekers. The research suggests a profound lack of immigrants' trust in Irish general practitioners (GPs) and outlines how formally sanctioned Western medicine fails these communities. The chapter points up some of the emerging consequences of globalisation in the form of economic migration and the problems physicians now face in dealing with increasing numbers of patients from diverse cultural backgrounds.

This raises issues of barriers to effective care for these communities and the consequences in terms of a failure in delivering appropriate and competent care. The authors discuss a 'heterogeneity of actions' within which utilisation of GP services is carefully negotiated and managed. They show that a range of heterodox health behaviours were drawn upon as alternatives or supplements to the use of GP services. These included the use of herbal treatments from health food shops and the use of informal lay networks to access familiar medicines from their home countries. Other strategies included describing symptoms over the telephone to family members or friends, or travelling to their home countries for medical treatment.

The chapter situates these findings in the broader literature about plural health practices in terms of culture and health, and pragmatism in health-seeking behaviour. In so doing it brings into sharp relief complex social and cultural issues that affect care in terms of competing health models and diverse treatment choices in an expanding pan-European (and now global) context. MacFarlane and de Brún emphasise the importance of multiple medical systems. Their discussion also brings us to complementary and alternative medicine, and the centrality of cultural ideas regarding health in terms of authenticity, allegiances and resistance to formal biomedicine, and they question the legitimacy of Western biomedicine as practised in the Irish context.

Their chapter emphasises medical pluralism and they begin by pointing up the variance within biomedicine(s) as 'culturally mediated practice', underlining Kleinman's point that biomedicine is an expression of a cultural system (Kleinman 1980). In so doing they draw attention to the limits of biomedicine. MacFarlane and de Brún underscore a central motif emerging in this volume, that of the pragmatic use of all available medical options (including biomedicine) rather than outright resistance to, or rejection of, biomedicine.

Part III explores policy implications and concentrates upon examining the distinction between folk healing and CAM, and also focuses on the regulation and ethical implications of folk medicine (Chapters 9, 10 and 11). In Chapter 9, Lee-Treweek emphasises the rise of the new healing markets and new forms of medical entrepreneurs. CAM has become big business in Western societies (McQuaide 2005). She illustrates how CAM, in its quest to complement biomedicine, is concerned with seeking professional recognition and formal legitimacy (within the biomedical model). Yet it uses a business approach similar to pyramid selling and often appears cult-like in its orientation. This raises important issues that separate CAM from traditional folk healing. These are issues of authenticity and commoditization, along with other tensions concerning training and apprenticeship (science) on the one hand and birth right (magic) on the other. She makes the point that social recognition (already pre-established for the folk healer) is often sought by CAM practitioners.

Lee-Treweek suggests that there is a basic flaw in the taxonomy used by serious writers in the field which has made the distinction between CAM and folk healing nebulous. Lee-Treweek suggests that this category error has permeated mainstream sociological thinking and has obscured an understanding of the true nature of folk medicine. Her chapter clarifies important distinctions between folk healers and CAM practitioners. This includes the tendency for CAM to be organised into separate modalities with boundaries and differentiation in terms of knowledge distribution and indemnity cover. It illustrates the professionalisation of complementary healing with an emphasis on credibility, knowledge base and proof of skills. She suggests that the rise and expansion of CAM in Britain has effectively undermined and annexed indigenous, traditional folk healers. Lee-Treweek argues that for CAM practitioners, monetary exchange is important in passing on skills of healing or access to healing. Others have shown this to be an important distinguishing feature between faith healers who have an international appeal and are more entrepreneurial, and folk healers (see Buckley 1980; Moore, this volume). The point here is that CAM is regarded as non-organic, appropriated, tied to modernity and contrived.

In Chapter 10, Stone considers the licensing, payment and legal position of folk healers and argues that there is partial recognition by the British Department of Health in moving some practices towards statutory regulation (under the auspices of the Medical Council). She argues that (with the exception of herbal medicines) folk healing has traditionally sat outside formal regulatory structures. As the rest of CAM moves towards greater professionalisation, and as non-U.K.

healing modalities become mainstream, questions arise as to whether indigenous folk healing could be, and should be, regulated – that is, restricted to those with 'appropriate' training and qualifications. There is particular concern in relation to 'the inappropriate healer' (see Moore, this volume) and 'the fraudulent healer' (Lee-Treweek, this volume).

Stone looks at pro- and anti-regulation positions. One of the arguments advanced is that failure to regulate may be harmful, so raising the issue of safety and quality assurance. Also, since CAM is now moving toward recognition and regulation, why shouldn't folk medicine? Stone raises the point that since healers know what they are doing they are potentially legally culpable under common law. This implies ethical expectations and appropriate ways of behaving, and, to this extent, the folk healer owes a duty of care. She makes the point that while the contemporary mantra is 'consumer choice', ill people remain potentially vulnerable. Alternatively, autonomy may be held to be important in a world where legally sanctioned and prescribed medicine and drugs have also been charged with having iatrogenic consequences.

Stone emphasises key points raised throughout the volume, arguing that folk healing is resistant to commoditisation precisely because formal regulation is incompatible with folk healing. In other words, the magic would be lost. The chapter suggests that more research is needed to explore the feasibility of alternative forms of, or basic measures of, regulation that could be adopted in folk healing, and advocates some form of formal licensing, using as an exemplar the Ontario model.

In the final chapter, McClean and Moore discuss contrasting perspectives that are instructive in explaining the changing boundaries between informal and formal healthcare. These discussions point to the changing and contested nature of healthcare and medicine in contemporary society; lay and professional health beliefs; and the juxtaposition of scientific and lay health practices. Finally, it pulls together key empirical and theoretical strands, and points towards an agenda for future applied research in health and medicine.

Notes

1. Cecil Helman's colourful account of his experiences as both anthropologist and general practitioner in *Suburban Shaman* (Helman 2006) is one of the notable exceptions.

References

Alver, B. 1981. 'Folk Medicine as an Open Medical System', in T. Vaskilampi and C. MacCormack (eds) *Folk Medicine and Health Culture:The Role of Folk Medicine in Modern Health Care*. Kuopio: Department of Community Health, University of Kuopio.

______. 1995. 'The Bearing of Folk Belief on Cure and Healing', *Journal of Folklore Research* 32(1): 21–33.

Bakx, K. 1991. 'The Eclipse of Folk Medicine in Western Society', *Sociology of Health and Illness* 13(1): 20–38.

Broom, A. and P. Tovey. 2007. 'The Dialectical Tension Between Individuation and Depersonalization in Cancer Patients' Mediation of Complementary, Alternative and Biomedical Cancer Treatments', *Sociology* 41(6): 1021–39.

Buckley, T. 1980. 'Unofficial Healing in Ulster', *Ulster Folklife* 26: 15–34.

Croom, E.M. 1992. 'Herbal Medicine Among the Lumbee Indians', in J. Kirkland, H.F. Mathews, C.W. Sullivan and K. Baldwin (eds), *Herbal and Magical Medicine*. Durham, NC: Duke University Press.

De Wert, E. 1984. 'Folk Healers as Part of Local Health Care System: A Case Study in Northern Norway', *Temenos* 20: 101–121.

Earwood, C. 1999. 'Trees and Folk Medicine', *Folk Life* 38: 22–31.

Evans-Pritchard, E.E. 1976. *Witchcraft, Oracles and Magic Among the Azande*, rev. edn. Oxford: Clarendon Press.

Gevitz, N. (ed.) 1988. *Other Healers: Unorthodox Medicine in America*. Baltimore, MD: John Hopkins University Press.

Hand, W.D. 1971. 'The Folk Healer: Calling and Endowment', *Journal of the History of Medicine* 26: 263–75.

______. 1980. *Magical Medicine*. Berkeley: University of California Press.

Hänninen, O. 1981. 'On the Physiology of the Healing Methods in Folk Medicine', in T. Vaskilampi and C. MacCormack (eds), *Folk Medicine and Health Culture: The Role of Folk Medicine in Modern Health Care*. Kuopio: Department of Community Health, University of Kuopio.

Helman, C.G. 1986. '"Feed a Cold, Starve a Fever"', in C. Currer and M. Stacey (eds), *Concepts of Health, Illness and Disease*. Oxford: Berg.

______. 2006. *Suburban Shaman: Tales from Medicine's Front Line*. London: Hammersmith Press.

Hufford, D.J. 1988. 'Contemporary Folk Medicine', in N. Gevitz (ed.) *Other Healers: Unorthodox Medicine in America*. Baltimore, MD: John Hopkins University Press.

______. 1992. 'Folk Medicine in Contemporary America', in J. Kirkland, H.F. Mathews, C.W. Sullivan and K. Baldwin (eds), *Herbal and Magical Medicine*. Durham, NC: Duke University Press.

______. 1997. 'Folk Medicine and Health Culture in Contemporary Society', *Complementary and Alternative Therapies in Primary Care* 24(4): 723–41.

Kaptchuk, T.J. and D.M. Eisenberg. 2001. 'Varieties of Healing, 2: A Taxonomy of Unconventional Healing Practices', *Annals of Internal Medicine* 135(3): 196–204.

Kirkland, J. 1992. 'Taking Fire Out of Burns: A Magico-religious Healing Tradition', in J. Kirkland, H.F. Mathews, C.W. Sullivan and K. Baldwin (eds), *Herbal and Magical Medicine*. Durham, NC: Duke University Press.

Kirkland, J., H.F. Mathews, C.W. Sullivan and K. Baldwin (eds). 1992. *Herbal and Magical Medicine*. Durham, NC: Duke University Press.

Kleinman, A. 1980. *Patients and Healers in the Context of Culture: An Exploration of the Borderland between Anthropology, Medicine and Psychiatry*. Berkeley: University of California Press.

Levine, H.D. 1941. 'Folk Medicine in New Hampshire', *New England Journal of Medicine* 224(12): 487–92.

McClean, S. 2003. 'Doctoring the Spirit: Exploring the Use and Meaning of Mimicry and Parody at a Healing Centre in the North of England', *Health: An Interdisciplinary Journal for the Social Study of Health, Illness and Medicine* 7(4): 483–500.

______. 2005. "The Illness is Part of the Person": Discourses of Blame, Individual Responsibility and Individuation at a Centre for Spiritual Healing in the North of England', *Sociology of Health and Illness* 27(5): 628–48.

MacCormack, C. 1981. 'Introduction: Traditional Medicine, Folk Medicine and Alternative Medicine', in T. Vaskilampi and C. MacCormack (eds), *Folk Medicine and Health Culture: The Role of Folk Medicine in Modern Health Care*. Kuopio: Department of Community Health, University of Kuopio.

McQuaide, M.M. 2005. 'The Rise of Alternative Health Care: A Sociological Account', *Social Theory and Health* 3(4): 286–301.

Mathews, H.F. 1987. 'Rootwork: Description of an Ethnomedical System: the American South', *Southern Medical Journal* 80: 885–91.

———. 1992. 'Introduction: A Regional Approach. In J. Kirkland, H.F. Mathews, C.W. Sullivan and K. Baldwin (eds) *Herbal and Magical Medicine*. London: Duke University Press.

Napolitano, V. and G.M. Flores. 2003. 'Complementary Medicine: Cosmopolitan and Popular Knowledge, and Transcultural Translations – Cases from Urban Mexico', *Theory, Culture and Society* 20(4): 79–95.

Press, I. 1978. 'Urban Folk Medicine: A Functional Overview', *American Anthropologist* 80: 71–84.

Scott, C.S. 1974. 'Health and Healing Practices Among Five Ethnic Groups in Miami, Florida', *Public Health Reports* 89(6): 524–32.

Snow, L.F. 1978. 'Sorcerers, Saints and Charlatans: Black Folk Healers in Urban America', *Culture, Medicine and Psychiatry* 2: 69–106.

Trotter, R.T. and J.A. Chavira. 1997. *Curanderismo: Mexican-American Folk Healing*, 2nd edn. Athens: University of Georgia Press.

Vaskilampi, T. 1981. 'Culture and Folk Medicine', in T. Vaskilampi and C. MacCormack (eds), *Folk Medicine and Health Culture: The Role of Folk Medicine in Modern Health Care*. Kuopio: Department of Community Health, University of Kuopio.

Chapter 2

Folk Healing and a Post-scientific World

Ronnie Moore and Stuart McClean

With us ther was a doctour of phisik;
In al this world ne was ther noon hym lik,
To speke of phisik and of surgerye,
For he was grounded in astronomye.
He kepte his pacient a ful greet deel
In houres by his magyk natureel.

–Geoffrey Chaucer, *The Canterbury Tales*

One day, a patient came in and told me, 'I don't take medicine.' Before I moved on, I asked, 'Do you take anything else?' She said, 'Oh yeah,' and pulled out a large bag of supplements – to which I replied, 'Well, so I see: If the FDA will approve it, you won't take it; but if they don't approve it, you will.' Then she laughed and said 'Well yeah, something like that.' What I considered medicine, she didn't.

–Lee Balance (2002)

Folk Healing as History, Revival and Rediscovery

Indigenous medicine and folk healing extend back to prehistory and yet are practised throughout the modern world to a greater or lesser degree. Charles Leslie summarised the legacy of ancient medical customs thus: 'The health concepts and practices of most people in the world today continue traditions that evolved during antiquity' (Leslie 1977: 1). Archaeology and physical anthropology have uncovered evidence of skills in primitive surgery (trephining), bone setting and early apothecary with the magico-medical use of plants, herbs, roots and berries (Broca 1876; Finger and Fernando 2001). The Egyptian Ebers Smith Papyrus, for example, makes reference to the importance of manipulation and the use of hands in traditional forms of therapy and documents some 876 prescriptions and 800 substances (Kaptchuk and Croucher 1987).

Magic, in the form of spells, charms and cures is also widely believed to have been a central feature of these early health care systems thousands of years before the rise of Christianity and biblical cures. Early traditional healing combined superstition (that which could not be explained) and science (tried and proven remedies and practices). These two seemingly opposing practices and ideologies were not as antithetical as they seem today. The links between religion, superstition, magic and science therefore need further elaboration and careful clarification.

As the term suggests, folk healing is tied to ecology, geography and local culture, and is based on 'traditional' beliefs (largely handed down via a process of oral communication and of socialisation): 'The tendency of many folklorists and anthropologists has been to seek for uniformity rather than a diversity of attitudes, beliefs and practices' (Graham 1985: 178). Folk healing in its widest sense refers to a matrix of multiple and culturally varied health belief systems, and sub-systems, throughout the world. These systems rest not on universal laws, but rather on a wide spectrum of specific 'organic' healing beliefs, traditions, powers and practices. These are by definition idiosyncratic, ethnocentric and culturally specific. They are tied to local contingencies and linked to pragmatically oriented world-views. There are as many different folk beliefs and practices, and health systems, as there are folk cultures in the world and this has tended to obviate an all-encompassing definition of folk healing or folk medicine. Comparability therefore is difficult because nomenclature is problematic.[1]

The folk healer may refer to persons who have acquired or have learnt about curative powers, medical or healing knowledge from experts, kin or local practitioners. Various titles commonly assigned to practitioners have included, but are not exclusive to, 'cunning man', 'wise woman', 'witch', 'witch doctor', 'shaman', 'medicine men', 'spirit healers' and more. Folk medicine or healing may involve a singular act, or combinations of curative skills or healing knowledge. Since healing practices are inextricably linked to localised and culturally specific expressions, incorporating religion, law and politics, it makes little sense to talk of folk healing or folk medicine as if it were a singular, unified or codified practice. Cultural variations therefore make categorisation problematic; it is not (nor could it be) a distinctly unified and codified system. This presents problems in terms of comparative analysis since such practices are representative of multiple healthcare systems: 'Even a cursory review of the literature on Comparative Health Systems (CHS) shows a vast array of models, criteria, concepts and critiques' (Whiteford and Nixon 2000: 440).

Common themes, however, do cut across cultures, leading to an attempt at some classification. Modern parlance has tended to homogenise terminology and practices. For example, within inter-disciplinary and cross-disciplinary health and social sciences there is increased talk of a variety of folk-healing movements; terms such as holistic, traditional, complementary and alternative, as well as fringe and marginal medicine, are commonly discussed in the literature. The classification 'alternative medicine' has been popular in the literature due to the practices' noted political marginality in the healthcare system. 'Alternative' denotes those practices not officially recognised or sanctioned by the state, which are alternative because of 'their socio-politically defined marginal standing in the health care system' (Saks 1992: 3).

Folk healing and folk medicine have long been viewed as a distrusted practice and in an increasingly modern, complex scientific-centric world have been cast aside, derided and banished. However, there is increasing recognition within disciplines like anthropology that the debate surrounding the relationship between such 'magical' practices and modernity is complex, multifaceted and as yet unresolved (Pels 2003). Nevertheless, popular ideas surrounding folk healing have for a considerable period assumed a lowly position compared to Western biomedicine or formal medicine, and as such have not had recourse to the hegemonic forms of authority and power that biomedicine takes refuge in. The discourse therefore often implies a power relationship with, and deference to, legitimate Western social and medical order.

In this chapter we seek to unearth the foundations of health and healthcare systems, beginning with basic ideas surrounding cosmology, religion and magic. This discussion develops historical explanations of health beliefs and practices, locating these within mainstream social science and historical literature. In so doing, we problematise received wisdom, demonstrating, for example, the centrality of subterranean folk beliefs and healing practices within modern Britain and Ireland. We recognise important historical and more contemporary ethnographic contributions on the European continent (see van Gennep 1937; Lindquist 2005; Quave and Pieroni 2005; see also Ramsey 1999). And we seek to provide further building blocks for cross-cultural comparison. In addition, we deal with a number of important connections, such as links between religion, superstition, magic and science. Finally, we discuss the rise and position of scientific medicine and the connections between biomedicine and folk medicine (folk healing as an alternative organic practice is considered in many ways equal to biomedicine).

Cosmology, Religion and Magic

Different cultures and societies in the world have tried to make sense of their existence in relation to their social and ecological circumstances, and have offered particular 'folk' explanations for health. These form part of elaborate cosmological and cosmogonical belief systems seeking to explain 'this world' events and experiences, including health and illness, with reference to deities, magic and religion.[2] These explanations may also be dysfunctional as well as functional (Mathews 1994). Animism – that is, the belief in the spirit or soul – may be regarded as a basic form of religion in primitive culture from which others have evolved (Tylor 1958[1871]). As Tambiah (1990) suggests, we must acknowledge a debt to Tylor because his seminal work provided an important starting point for serious intellectual discussions of religion. Although Tylor's evolutionary ideas are thought to be problematic, his concept of animism may not so easily be dismissed (Lambek 2002).[3] 'Anthropology still needs an adequate theory of belief, and with his emphasis on thought processes, Tylor, I suggest, might offer us one possibility for developing such a theory' (Stringer 1999: 547).

In premodern and traditional societies, beliefs about health and illness were socially and morally tied to ideas of good and evil, the sacred and profane (Turner 2000: 9). It was believed that malevolent forces (natural and supernatural) might be harnessed or controlled. The healing arts and malevolent practices fall within this spectrum.

Sanders, for example, using wide ranging ethnographic examples, discusses illness, infant mortality and influenza epidemics and their connection with the idea of the witch. He illustrates that belief in witchcraft was common worldwide among a great number and variety of cultures and societies (Sanders 1995: 10–29). Witches were thought to possess a magical ability to cause, diagnose and control misfortune and illness. Witches could be blamed for illness, such as rheumatism, arthritis and strokes. No specific illness or disease was always blamed on witchcraft, although strange, unidentifiable and inexplicable diseases were particularly likely to be attributed to witches (ibid.: 34). The link with health and well-being is explicit and the terms 'witch' and 'doctor' are interchangeable in the literature (ibid.) The witch phenomenon later impacted on the persecution of (usually marginalised) groups and individuals, and continues to influence contemporary health issues (Sanders 1995; La Fontaine 1998).

Folk-healing practices are tied to 'otherworldly', magical and religious beliefs, in terms of ways of seeing the world, and also in terms of individual and collective action and organisation resulting from this. These 'sacred canopies' essentially attempted to explain mystical and magical ideas that in a precarious and dangerous world could not be readily understood, conceptualised, or explained, such as sickness and death, good and evil, fortune and misery: 'God has also chosen certain men and women and given them powers to control the devil. Curanderos are healers par excellence with powers of divination. They are helpful not only in cases of illness, but also in instances of bewitchment that result in bad luck, matrimonial problems, alcoholism, and any number of other problems' (Graham 1985: 170). The connections between magic, religion, good fortune and health, social organisation and disorganisation are expressed in the classic social science literature. The social, functional aspects of magic and religion and the consequences for social organisation and social behaviour, for example, were major themes in early sociological and anthropological texts (Mauss and Hubert 1972[1902]; Frazer 1911; Durkheim 1976[1915]; Rivers 2001[1924]; Evans-Pritchard 1937). These looked at 'religion'; that is, shared spiritual beliefs and formalised institutional bodies that seek to make sense of worldly and otherworldly domains and connect the living and the dead. They also discussed 'the social' in defining, understanding and reifying the role, place and significance of 'other worldly', spiritual ideas and shared cosmological beliefs. Durkheim's *The Elementary Forms of Religious Life* (Durkheim 1976[1915]) was centrally concerned with human 'collective conscience' rather than God. Malinowski (1974[1948]) viewed belief systems as means of providing structure and predictability for uncertain and dangerous contexts. To this end, magico-religious healing and reference to deities provided systems of coping with illness, death and the unknown (Turner 2000).

But religion is a complex and multifaceted concept. It is, as Tylor (1958[1871]) suggests, a belief in spiritual beings, but it is also symbolic practice, group organisation and institution (Hamilton 2005: 18). Religion appears at once to be sacred and profane, individual and collective, social cement and social division, social restriction and social capital. Religion is the theistic or metaphysical character of spirituality that often seeks to provide an explanation for existence. But it also provides explicit rules (and sanctions) for living. As such, religion and religious beliefs act as an important organising principle. It represents a common moral integrative value system, with institutions, symbolic rituals, rites and ceremonies. Religion is 'a unified system of beliefs and practices relative to sacred things, that is to say, things set apart and forbidden – beliefs and practices which unite into one single moral community called a church, all those who adhere to them' (Durkheim 1976: 47).

For Durkheim religion was 'the social collective'; for Weber it was 'moral individualism' and subjectivism (*sola fide*). Both principles are central to debates concerning the traditional and the modern, superstition and science, and, as a consequence, to seemingly competing health paradigms in the Western world: 'I believe that we should regard the Protestant reformation as not only one source of modernization, but also its defence against magic, superstition, witchcraft or mysticism. Calvinistic Protestantism was crucial in the development of modern forms of individuality, rationalism, and asceticism; it generated and preserved many of the essential features of what we mean by the notion of modernity' (Turner 1991: xvii). Weber's Protestant ethic thesis explored a phase of the emancipation from magic (Bendix 1966: 69). In this he described 'the inner loneliness afflicting Calvinists as the culmination of a process that had been initiated by Hebrew prophets and fostered by Hellenistic science, a process which eliminated magic from the world; salvation and redemption could no longer be found through the magic of the church' (Kassell 2005a: 45).

Scholars have argued that by the mid seventeenth century the world had become individualised and 'disenchanted'. The observed changes prompted many (including Comte, Marx, Durkheim, Weber and Evans-Prichard) to speculate, further, that theistic aspects of religion would wane as modern society became increasingly scientific and rational (Comte's 'positive' phase of human history). Indeed, religion as a belief system appeared to be critically undermined throughout the nineteenth century as evolutionary and anthropological theories were set against theological doctrine.

Magical Monopoly

Supernatural beliefs and magical practice (including witchcraft) are generally seen as being tied to a particular historical past, located in a pre-industrial, premodern world, or in exotic tribal societies. Magic, as the container for a wider conceptual field incorporating shamanism, witchcraft, occultism and totemism, was widely perceived as the antithesis of modernity, 'a production of illusion and delusion that was thought to recede and disappear as rationalization and secularization spread throughout society' (Pels 2003: 4). A universal definition of magic is problematic, not least because magical beliefs and ritual tend to be culturally specific and may not be easily recognised. Magic is, however, believed to involve heterogeneous mystical practices. Only after the sixteenth century (in England) was it common to homogenise these as 'magic'. The Church saw magic as the unauthorised and diabolical attempt to manipulate the supernatural, 'including any folk practices previously regarded by their adherents as godly' (Thomas 1975: 97). The historical connection between healing, medicine and magic are extensively documented. Kassell, for example, describes how, in 1625, the French medical student Naudé wrote a history of magic identifying four specific types associated with god, angels, demons and human industry. This detailed natural magic and its application in mechanics and in medicine (Kassell 2006: 112).

Christianity (based on a messianic belief and universal principles) spread northwards throughout Eastern and Western Europe and replaced the notion of multiple anima and local deities with the belief in the one true God and the promise of an afterlife for those compliant or for those deemed worthy. In so doing it has aided in the demise of ancient supernatural ideas and traditional healing practices. Yet, paradoxically, Christianity has provided a continued rationale and basis for supernatural belief. Christian doctrine itself is contradictory, not least because of the belief in the Holy Trinity. It also includes 'mystery cults' and involves the holy communion of the faithful with God through progressive ritualised acts from baptism to burial, some of which are symbolic of cannibalism. We may add other aspects to this including devotion to preferred saints (depending on occasion or personal needs), the special or magical properties of holy water, holy pictures, relics, amulets, statues, prayer beads (thought to be an import from the Middle East by returning Crusaders) and associated paraphernalia (see Blackman 1918). Christianity itself enforced specific forms of magical belief and in so doing created a monopoly of magic and supernatural beliefs.

The bible teaches us about Christ the healer. This image is further enhanced in the writings of Saint Ambrose and Saint Augustine. We also see healing attributed to Saint Francis of Assisi, and later (and perhaps more uncomfortable) accounts of miraculous healing from others, such as Marie-Bernarde Soubirous (Saint Bernadette) and, more recently, modern faith healers including Benny Hinn. The distinction is made between religiously sanctioned (lawful) magic and that which was not sanctioned (unlawful magic). Christianity explicitly banished lay or occult magical practices. Pre-Christian, pagan and druidic beliefs emphasised multiple deities, revered nature, and were sourced from the immediate local environment. These were significant belief systems common in Britain, Ireland and much of Western Europe. The Roman Emperor Constantine, however, decreed that Christianity be made the official religion of the Empire. Pagan worship was banned under threat of death. As the geographic map of the Roman Empire expanded, and as Roman law began to dominate, pagan beliefs waned as Christianity began its ascendancy in Europe, yet the demise was never complete. Traditional Pagan healing practices, however, remained as survivals within the new religious order. As Porter suggests: 'Early Christianity exhibits a medley of attitudes towards healing shaping fluid relations between medicine and the church. Many old healing practices were dressed up in new Christian garbs; Christian shrines were raised upon the ruins of pagan temples and the leading healing saints, Cosmas and Damian, were in some respects revampings of the heathen Castor and Pollux' (Porter 1998: 86). The rise of Christianity exposed multiple communal and personal tensions. On the one hand it forcibly banished traditional indigenous belief systems and localised magical practice, yet it continually referenced biblical miracles or cures. Out of this schizophrenic attitude emerged the text of two Dominican monks, *Malleus Maleficarum*, which 'shows that even at the height of the Renaissance and at the threshold of the Reformation, the conflict between paganism and Christianity, between magic and a more enlightened monolithic outlook, had not ceased to be a burning issue in more than one sense of the word. The ancient idols and deities, torn down from their pedestals a long time ago, had not altogether lost their grip on men's minds' (Ehrenwald (1956: 114–15). Visits to holy places, holy wells, shrines and sites of apparitions – such as Lourdes (France), Fátima (Portugal) and Knock (Ireland) – self-harm in Mediterranean Catholic villages such as Guardia Sanframondi (Italy), or miracles associated with the cult of the European Black Madonna (believed to have grown out of pre-Christian earth-goddess traditions; see Benko 1993), continually emphasise the centrality of magic and the supernatural in Christianity.

Magical sentiment is also embedded in modernity; indeed, it could be said to be *of* modernity rather than opposed to it (see Pels 2003). Superstition remains deeply rooted in our psyche and influences behaviour and decision making. Even if one does not personally adhere to such beliefs and practices, others around us do, and behaviour may be in accordance with such beliefs. Black cats crossing our path, not walking on cracks in a footpath, the number thirteen, avoiding walking under ladders, the colour green, wearing a rabbit's foot, sigils or amulets such as Saint Christopher medals, first footers (whereby people with red hair are prevented from being the first to cross a threshold in a new year) are symbolic representations of this. Superstition even pervades language: the German noun *Glück* refers both to happiness and luck.

Christian asceticism and the Protestant Reformation further attacked traditional pagan or heathen beliefs (and what they saw as the remnants of these in Catholicism) as Calvinist ideology imposed a new kind of spiritual, moral, social and cognitive order in Europe:

> The apostles instituted and left behind them water, oil, salt and lights to signify great mysteries. 'Papists' did not understand that these things were signifiers, not signs, and worshipped them idolatrously as though they were inherently holy. They invented other false practices outright. The reformers cast away these signs, mistaking them for superstitions, and these ceremonies were at the heart of the current division of the church. (Kassell 2006: 116)

The distinction between magic and religion was originally formulated by the sixteenth-century Protestant reformers who reinterpreted magic as coercive (Thomas 1975: 96; Tambiah 1990). English Protestantism thus marked a distinctive period from medieval England and its reliance on Catholic theology: 'If the distinction between magic and religion had been blurred by the medieval church, it was strongly reasserted by the propagandists of the Protestant Reformation' (Tambiah 1990: 18). Witchcraft persecutions were at their height around the 1580s. Estes suggests that in the period leading up to the seventeenth century it was common for the clergy to practice medicine (medical knowledge advancement was also intrinsically bound up with the monasteries), and there is sufficient historical evidence suggesting that practitioners diagnosed a disease as having been caused by a witch (Estes 1983: 275). Religion and medicine were both horsemen in the hunt for 'the witch'. Papists and Reformers alike persecuted to eliminate the threat and contamination of witchcraft and magic. The most famous examples include the Inquisition in Europe and the witch finders in New England.

New inventions also had an impact on belief and behaviour. The printing press facilitated the rapid expansion of more austere, Christian guiding principles. This may also have had a public-health function, as disease was considered as retribution for those who failed to adhere to God's laws. It is extremely likely that the diffusion of Puritanism was a consequence of the spread of syphilis in Europe: 'God's punishment for the sins of men' (Andreski 1980: 79).

Disenchantment or Amnesia?

The official history of indigenous or traditional folk healing shows that ancient belief systems were in decline, banished to the periphery and to the absurd: 'many Western philosophers are concerned with how early Greek thought ... was transformed from "magic" to "science," and ... the seeds sown by the Greek Philosophers ultimately flowered in the scientific revolution of the seventeenth century' (Lambek 2002: 345). However, magic and magical practices were not, as some historians and sociologists have suggested, neatly replaced by rationality. The well-known British historian Keith Thomas (1973), following Weber, suggested that the world has become 'disenchanted'. Natural laws came to replace the Aristotelian and neo-Platonist scholastic traditions; the rise of science was thought to erode the world of magic.

The pre-industrial sixteenth and seventeenth centuries represented a precarious and hazardous world with high rates of mortality and morbidity. Death was less predictable than it is today. Death and disease were personally close to individuals, families and whole communities. Crop failure and pestilence meant that many were susceptible to illness, starvation and the elements. This is exemplified by one of the worst scourges in terms of its virulence and proportion, the Black Death. Arriving in England in 1348, it is believed to have killed between a third, possibly up to a half of the population in England by the close of the century.

The disenchantment thesis argues that belief in magic declined in the post-Reformation period. However, this thesis, famously developed by Thomas, and detailed as it was, did not stack up on a number of counts. For example, medieval theologians and the Lollard mumblers of the mid fourteenth century (predating the Reformation) expressed self-help and rationalist tendencies. The notion that the decline of magic enabled the rise and expansion of technology was problematic. As Clark has shown, intellectual magic did not run counter to science (Clark 1997). In other words, Thomas could not readily explain the decline in magic as he had thought.

The thesis is not supported by recent historical evidence either. Kassell, in her analysis of Elizabethan London, for example, illustrates in some detail the continued existence and importance of magic in the city, the very place where you might expect rationality to succeed superstition. Magic and the belief in magic were actually thriving in Elizabethan London, even among physicians, and Kassell (2005b) illustrates how magic, religion, science and medicine were tightly intertwined. Thomas concedes that 'the sectarians', because of their emphasis on prophecy and religious healing, returned much of the magic that the reformers had rejected back to religion (Thomas 1975: 96). 'Pentecostal churches reject traditional culture, but also have a supernaturalistic vision of reality, with a discourse of God and the Devil, miraculous interventions, and an instrumental understanding of religion, all of which accords with aspects of traditional thinking, including the dynamics of witchcraft' (Bowie 2006: 228). In reality, tensions between Christianity, in its various denominational guises, and the traditional pre-Christian order were mediated, because multiple belief systems emerged that incorporated both religious and traditional magical beliefs.

Right up until the late eighteenth century, healing practices were multiplex and cannot be said to have been fully monopolised or dominated by any single professional group. Rather those who offered curative and health services included a variety of individuals. This included, barber-surgeons, physicians, various forms of druggists, apothecaries and alchemists, and an assortment of street-corner empirics and local healers (Ehrenreich and English 1972: 6–7; Porter 1993). The role of women as healers and managers of healthcare in the domestic setting was rarely acknowledged (many had formerly acted as empirics). The legacy of biblical teaching, witchcraft and the role of women in patriarchal Europe preserved their subordinate position and their virtual invisibility.

Up until the 1790s a complex array of healing knowledge, practices and products flourished in Europe (Bynum and Porter 1987; Harrison 1987; Neve 1987; Porter 1993; Lawrence 1994). This situation had implications for the way that so-called folk and what have been called 'fringe' practices and miracle cures were perceived: 'Treating and caring for the sick was no one's monopoly' (Lawrence 1994: 7). Indeed, Friedman (1981) discusses how in eighteenth-century France there was perceived to be little difference between the meaning of physician and that of healer; later this division became one of physician and quack.[4] A form of 'pluralism' in medicine existed in Europe during this time; diversity in health-seeking behaviour even among monarchs was the norm. Witness the influence of significant and influential historical figures such as Rasputin, for example.

However, one has to be careful in presenting a historical image of folk-healing practices as having particularly 'ancient' roots and therefore competing somehow on a level playing field with biomedical treatments during this relatively narrow period of European history. Although many folk practices did predate the modern period, many others sprang up and evolved during the same period of expansion in biomedical knowledge in the nineteenth century. As Bakx explains, folk healing and medicine is not just about the past, it is contemporary: 'Many folk practices are contemporaneous with much of biomedical practice. They were developed, not in some pre-modern past, but in the same nineteenth-century crucible from which sprang 'science' in general and biomedicine in particular' (Bakx 1991: 28).

Medical pluralism has always been a feature in Western societies in one form or another (Wallis and Morley 1976; Bakx 1991; Cant and Sharma 1999). A choice between formal and informal medicine has always existed and, despite a short period of 'eclipse', the state of the health services is again in a period of plurality (Bakx 1991). Contemporary folk-inspired healing practices are not primarily a residual category of a pre-Enlightenment period (ibid.: 28). The contemporary situation symbolises the 'resurgence' of healing practices, but many of these practices are distinct from those that were common during the eighteenth century. A distinction therefore between premodern medical pluralism and the 'new' medical pluralism of industrial capitalism is a useful one (Cant and Sharma 1999). Frankenberg (1980) has asserted medical pluralism is an inevitable feature of class-divided societies. We would concur with that; pluralism has always been extant in European society, and is unlikely to diminish in the foreseeable future.

Magical Efficacy

Popular ideology suggests that science and rationality, what we might call modernity, appears to have unmasked and exposed magic and, in so doing, has usurped its prominence. The spells are forgotten, the cordials subjected to spectrometry, the incantations banished to 'mumbo jumbo' and the amulets hidden. In the modern world folk healing has been marginalised and stigmatised as odd, mystical and irrational; in contrast, biomedical practitioners are 'arch-modernity personified' (Bakx 1991: 30). The 'folk' is associated with our primitive past.

Part of the problem is the lack of appreciation of the indigenous nature of folk medicine. It is often based on local organic practices not fully understood outside their immediate socio-cultural and cognitive frameworks. Industrialisation and urbanisation changed the context of traditional social life, pulling people away from the traditional agrarian matrix (of local culture and belief systems) into a new modernised world that raised expectations and promised much beyond that which it could deliver.

Folk medicine and magical beliefs are not simply survivals in a modern age, but are a necessary and integral part of healthcare systems in the West. As such they need to be understood in terms of their functions for individuals who adhere to them, and in terms of their function for society. Anthropologists tend to emphasise the symbolic character and social functions of magic as the real rationale behind the practice (Hamilton 2005: 38), in addition to recognising the historicity of our knowledge claims (Good 1994). Magico-religious beliefs and practices act as agents of social control. They are tied to moral responsibility (Durkheim 1976[1915]) and provide rules for social interaction in all kinds of situations (Evans-Pritchard 1937). These have both manifest and latent relevance. Local people themselves emphasise the actual efficacy of folk medicine. Magical beliefs may not be empirical claims, but this does not mean that they are without powers that have real, concrete and material effects (Hamilton 2005: 9): 'Primitive medicine is primarily magico-religious, utilizing a few rational elements while our (modern scientific) medicine is predominantly rational and specific, employing a few magic elements' (Ackerknect 1946: 475).

Bowie reminds us that, 'Philosophers and theologians ... have argued for the rationality of believing in God, and supposedly irrational beliefs, such as witchcraft, may appear to be supported by empirical evidence' (Bowie 2006: 226). In *The Science of Magic*, for example, Coe provides a convincing array of examples that suggest scientific explanation for the effects of magic, just as science can now explain much of the effects of some forms of 'alternative medicine'. Ulett, for example, has detailed the neurochemical and neuroanatomical evidence for explaining how acupuncture works (Ulett 1992, cited in Coe 1997: 3). Coe argues that many folk remedies are empirically correct, even if the understanding surrounding them may appear scientifically irrelevant. The debate however lies beyond the empirical: 'To be on the transcendental side was to think that natural science was not the last word – that there was more truth to be found. To be on the empirical side was to think that natural science – facts about how spatiotemporal things worked – was all the truth there was' (Rorty 1987: 29).

In highlighting the significance of the historicist turn, that 'truth is made and not found' (truth as socially constructed, as opposed to natural and innate), philosophers such as Richard Rorty have sought to free us from the binds of theology and metaphysics, and at the same time allow us to see the contextual, historical and contingent nature of knowledge systems (see Rorty 1989). Heavily critical of the Enlightenment, although not the sentiment, where 'science is no more than the handmaiden of technology' (ibid.: 3), such a conceptual scheme offers a way of locating the dominance of medical knowledge and the ways in which such knowledge has been 'naturalised' in Western societies. It is, according to Good, difficult and perhaps counter-intuitive to be relativist about the nature of disease and medicine. And yet, how do we accept this with our 'recognition of our own historicity and our desire to respect competing knowledge claims of members of other societies or status groups' (Good 1994: 3).

The Emergence of Formal Medicine and Professionalism

We are reminded that modern medical and health services were inspired by and emerged from monastic institutions. The rise and development of hospitals were a direct result of religious orders. Indeed, by the eighteenth century and the foundation of the hospitals, corporeal satisfaction ('this worldly' happiness) was no longer perceived as a sinful activity. Relaxation of the ideologies surrounding the importance of material pleasure led, *inter alia*, to the pursuit of health (Lawrence 1994). Early medical establishments cared for and healed both the body and the soul (Lane 2001). The curative process was itself a trinity, in the form of a magico-religious and medical event. This was the case in Europe, although the dissolution of the monasteries (1537) in England meant that sparse medical services afforded by the Church had virtually vanished. While medicine was born in the Church it was raised in the army.

The relationship between science and religion was complex. Celestial consultation was common in the medieval period. As long as astrology and astronomy did not contradict its teachings, the Church did not object. 'Zodiac man', referenced in numerous medieval medical manuscripts, is illustrative of the connection between astrology and medicine.

Even today, both family and Church retain their vital role as providers of health and social services alongside formal medicine. Religious faith was not threatened by science; early science was there to reveal the work of God. Even the early-modern philosopher Pierre Gassendi's (1592–1655) empiricism was influenced by his adherence to central teachings of Christian doctrine. That which could not be explained (including punctuated and mysterious evolution patterns and the various formulations and puzzles of the periodic table) was accounted for as 'the god of the gaps' – it was simply not yet revealed.

Even modern medical practitioners may or may not accept spirituality and religion in conjunction with their scientific beliefs. Like the sixteenth-century physician Andreas Vesalius before him, for the Africanist, physican and clergyman David Livingstone, the spiritual and the rational were not incongruous. Paracelsus was known to have been interested in astrology, chemistry and magic: 'he believed that within man there burned a primal spiritual urge, to be tapped in faith healing, in prayer, and in "the power of the word," that simply by describing illness or death, healing and the relief of pain could be induced' (Kaptchuk and Croucher 1987: 78).

Medicine had been based on a mixture of Galenic and Paracelsian chemical remedies and was practised by a small group of individuals.

By the early nineteenth century a recognisable medical profession had emerged. Formalised medical practice, with its particular brand of seventeenth-century Cartesian analytic philosophy, began to grow, though in Britain it did not come to dominate Western healthcare until after the establishment of the 1858 parliamentary act which established a medical register listing those allowed to formally use the appellation 'doctor' (even though the title refers to the highest rank of an academic degree). At the top, physicians were normally university educated, usually having studied only non-medical subjects such as philosophy; they advised patients, suggested remedies, and charged high fees. Surgeons had separated from the barbers in 1540, and were trained by a traditional apprenticeship; they carried out manual tasks, such as amputations and lancing boils. Apothecaries, also apprenticed, dispensed and sold medicines, often in their shops; the most numerous of medical practitioners, they were allowed to charge only for the pills or powders they dispensed, not for the advice they usually provided (Lane 2001: 1).[5]

However, even after the surgeons, apothecaries and physicians combined and established the beginnings of formal medicine, the initial clientele was not the masses. Instead, formal medicine treated those who could best afford it. Personal and financial desperation in seeking a cure or treatment and the difficulty of getting the services of a physician, surgeon or apothecary in the early part of the eighteenth century led to a thriving alternative market. Lane notes a separate industry of unqualified practitioners who marketed their activities, the empirics, who 'travelled the provinces to promote their cure' (ibid.: 8). When epidemics struck (leprosy, smallpox and typhus were common in the medieval period) formal medicine was largely ineffective, and people resorted to unqualified empirics or quacks (ibid.: 1).

The emergence of scientific rationalism, and the growth, expansion and dominance of formal medicine throughout the twentieth century, essentially imposed itself structurally on modern life, and psychologically on modern thinking. A range of heterodox folk medicines also grew during this period of rapid social and industrial change; as Porter (1993) explains, there was an appetite for medicines in general, which was not impeded by growing affluence and secularisation. However, formal medicine was becoming consolidated, basing itself on biological understandings of the body developed from Cartesian principles. Scientific 'discoveries' (Harvey and Lister are but two examples of prominent discoverers, although these discoveries may be sourced to much earlier periods in other parts of the world) appeared to hold a more elevated status (rather than public health discoveries, for example), and were continually adding to the biological 'scientific' knowledge base.

Science began to identify specific diseases throughout the nineteenth century and this led to the emergence of medical specialities. Concepts of disease began to change and this heralded the rise of the learned physician. In the new biomedical field, practitioners began to enjoy increasing social and economic status; at the same time, the role of folk healers and folk medicine was attacked. 'Most qualified practitioners considered that quacks threatened their professional livelihoods and sought to discredit them although often employing their techniques and even the same basic ingredients' (Lane 2001: 9).

The medical profession developed a highly professionalised organisational structure, which included important institutions of learning. It was becoming progressively more uncomfortable with religion and its associated baggage. The rational, objective, empirical, observable, testable and replicable were new mantras for a modernity that did not seek to reference the old order with its ancient practices. Rather, formal medicine's gaze focused on the body and its interior, and with scientific progress came a myopic focusing down on the organ, cell, atom, sub-atomic and now nuclear particle. Holistic medicine became much less important as medical training constantly emphasised biological science. The pipe smoking, family practitioner with detailed local knowledge who offered much more than a clinical service, as Porter suggests, was passing into history (Porter 1998).

However, attending a physician was not solely dependent on financial ability. It was not only the poor and uneducated that utilised folk medicine as a direct result of their impoverished circumstances. The wealthy and the nobility made use of folk healing also. Recent research indicates that when it comes to health, middle-class angst appears to have motivated the educated, fully acculturated and economically secure to pursue non-medical forms of healing (McQuaide 2005). There is an assumption that people use one healthcare system exclusively. The historical and empirical evidence suggests, however, that this is not the case. Alternative healing has been and is juxtaposed alongside, always acting as a corrective to, the limitations of formal medicine. Also, astute physicians are aware of the potency of 'the social' in the medical encounter:

> Mexican miners liked and respected Dr Wilson, the company doctor, and came to him with a great variety of complaints.... 'Well,' he said, 'Nine tenths of the people [Mexican] who came to see me for a treatment are really not in need of medicine at all, but if I don't prescribe something, they feel that I have no interest in them, or do not understand their case, and consequently will lose confidence in me. So I give them some non-medicated tablets with directions to take one after each meal, one at bedtime, and tell them if they don't get to feeling better in a few days to come back. If they return, I change the color of them and in a few days they will get well and I get the credit'. (cited in Graham 1985: 175–76)

Folk medicine was not something that people simply turned to in desperation when medical efforts were failing (McGuire and Kantor 1987: 221–22).

Despite assistance from the legal system and the state, formal biomedicine has never achieved absolute governance over healthcare and we suggest that its longer-term, future hegemony is not guaranteed. For example, during the Victorian period, a time when formal medicine was consolidating its interests, people maintained an interest and fascination in magical enchantments, from rites and spells to the Romantic movement – influenced by the writings and imaginings of Poe, Stoker and Mary Shelley (who cites the German alchemist and astrologer Agrippa in her works) – and to forms of occultism and spiritualism, all of which arguably reflected a period of 'high bourgeois anxiety' (Pels 2003: 9). And yet, despite the persistence of a diverse array of alternative and folk-inspired therapies, formal medicine's formally sanctioned position has not, as yet, been significantly challenged (Saks 1994), and the most likely scenario for the near future is the continued dominance of the medical profession (Saks 2001: 129).

The emergence of the hospital, and the emphasis on laboratory science as its knowledge base (Salmon 1984; Kelleher, Gabe and Williams 1994; Cant and Sharma 1999), were two key factors behind biomedicine's rise to dominance.[6] Beyond this, a variety of interlinking processes also led to its hegemonic position. These included secularisation in modern society, philanthropic tendencies in medicine, and the healthcare shift from 'care' to 'cure' (Stacey 1988).

The support and legitimacy that derive from biomedicine's association with the state has also been emphasised. Easthope (1986), for example, describes how core members of the medical profession during the late eighteenth and early nineteenth century formed a social group in London that established contact with the political elite. This led to various parliamentary health acts which secured biomedicine's formally sanctioned position, and had the subsequent effect of disengaging it from other practices which were equally prevalent at the time (Cant and Sharma 1999; Saks 1991). From another perspective, Lupton argues that biomedicine's dominance was established through its emphasis on science's association with authoritative expert knowledge (Lupton 1994: 107–8).

Gevitz (1988) also points to the advent of medical sectarianism during the nineteenth century, which was seen as partly a response to the medical profession's marshalling of its support, but also as a way of ensuring 'newly alternative' practices were increasingly organised. The more 'organised' and institutionalised practices – such as osteopathy, chiropractics and homeopathy – sought professional status so as to set themselves aside from other practices perceived as 'quackery'.

Biomedical dominance, professionalisation and elitism have meant that medical practitioners occupy a high occupational status and have been able to command high rewards. Salaries for this occupational group are already at an all-time high and physicians are influential well beyond the bounds of their discipline. The cultural gap between biomedical practitioners and their patients that Chaucer and Bakx (1991) allude to has become increasingly visible in recent times.

Today we see a conflict of interests where products and profits on the one hand, and care and services on the other, collide. Ireland, for example, emerged as one of the richest nations in the European Union and yet it retained an unenviable record in terms of healthcare compared with other member nations. The recent move to business models in the provision of healthcare in Britain has sparked concern that some physicians may be enhancing their incomes by exploiting the National Health Service's (NHS) internal market. In Britain, the NHS's new 'practice-based commissioning' scheme means that treatments may now be outsourced to private companies, and doctors can recommend these to patients. An investigation for Channel 4's news programme recently documented that in Liverpool, seventy-three physicians were shareholders of one private company that had won such a bid.[7]

Medicine's institutional authority is affected by a consumer-driven healthcare environment (Kaptchut and Eisenberg 2001). As the printing press brought the 'true' word of God and the Reformation to the masses (and launched the modern era of medicine), the World Wide Web brought with it access to knowledge, including medical knowledge, and demystified esoteric medical wisdom. In a postmodern or late-modern world, knowledge and information are democratised (Hardey 1999), and in seeking health information this brings benefits as well as risks (Hesse et al. 2005). In partial recognition of the problems facing current practitioners, medical pedagogy has reintroduced basic elements from the social sciences and the humanities in medical training. Critical observers would argue, however, that serious pedagogic engagement is limited and not fully considered in terms of planning or effectiveness.

The medical establishment slavishly pursues science. In truth, experienced physicians recognise the limits of modern medicine but most remain dismissive (to their peers at least) of 'marginal medicine'. Even the most disillusioned and alienated are compelled to remain in post because doctors have invested many years in training (and acculturation) to be professionals and are locked into a high-status lifestyle that requires a high salary. The status quo is maintained.

Folk Medicine and a Post-scientific World: From 'Eclipse' to Revitalisation

A division is drawn between official scientific rhetoric and pragmatic practice. Alternative medical practices have co-existed with formal scientific medicine. Indeed the relationship is symbiotic and there is a tacit recognition of this by many physicians and the lay community at large, which serves to illustrate a codependence of each. However, a 'modern scientific cosmology fails to offer an integrated model of the world that incorporates the values of both human beings and the eco system' (Bowie 2006: 115).

Keith Bakx (1991) highlights 'the eclipse of folk medicine' in Western society, making the point that folk medicine is firmly located within modern, late-modern or postmodern society, and not simply a survival from some pre-scientific past. Bakx questions whether the process of modernity, diverse and overwhelming as it is, has automatically led to the decline of folk practices:

> In Western society, it is generally assumed that folk practices have more or less died out. The eclipse of folk medicine is put on a par with the decline of religion and the demise of the community. That is to say, it is seen as being inversely proportional to the index of urbanisation or modernisation, themselves 'self-evident' measures of the development of capitalism. (ibid.: 21)

And yet, folk medical practices have not been eclipsed; rather, they have been transformed, revitalised and given new impetus: 'Folk medicine, like religiosity and community, has been transformed, but not eradicated by, the modernist project' (ibid.: 21). Some social theorists have adopted terms like postmodernity and late-modernity to provide an overarching conceptual framework with which to explain a general socio-cultural shift in Western societies.[8]

The social theorist Zygmunt Bauman (1995), for instance, argues that under modernity, identity, expressions of individuality and the formation of community were stable and fixed. Under these social conditions the individual had little room to manoeuvre between different and sometimes opposing 'life-worlds'. In postmodernity, (or late-modernity) these social relations and notions of belonging are loose and disposable. Identity and expressions of individuality become a 'DIY' creation: it is individually crafted and fashioned to the personal project.

Postmodernity, moreover, can be viewed as characterised by the privileging of subjectivity; indeed, these socio-cultural conditions represent an increasing trend towards a plurality of subjective discourses. In his analysis of postmodernity, Smart argues, 'We find ourselves living amidst a plurality of doctrines and styles of reasoning' (Smart 1993: 120), which highlights the particular ambiguity of the status of any particular knowledge claims, whether expert-defined or lay/folk. The implications for the status of scientific knowledge are outlined by Giddens: 'The post-modern outlook sees a plurality of heterogeneous claims to knowledge, in which science does not have a privileged place' (Giddens 1990: 2). Although science is the most culturally embedded and reflexive system of knowledge in modern society, we note that changes to the public status of science have fundamental implications for the legitimacy of knowledge in the postmodern era. The increasing importance of 'lay' or folk knowledge in Western societies is testament to that.

Saks continues this theme: postmodernity 'is normally conceived as being characterised by a plurality of cultures of social groups, with a tolerance of minorities and a willingness to combine multiple discourses' (Saks 1998: 203). This sentiment is echoed by Thompson, who explains that newly established forms of social identity and social groups, 'represent new and often surprising combinations and crossovers of codes and discourses' (Thompson 1992: 247). Therefore, new social groups seek to combine the institutional features of modernity alongside those values that seem to have been hitherto excluded. For example: 'The kinds of phenomena include some that modernist thought would have regarded as marginal or antithetical to modern life: the sacred, charisma, passion, spirituality, cosmic meaning and unity, enchantment, community' (ibid.)

In a similar vein, Beck (1992) asserts that we live in a risk-laden world as risks are an intrinsic and ever expanding part of modern life. We now live in an age of advanced modernity and, according to Beck, technological risk is part of this age. Mary Douglas similarly considers risk in modern Western society, in particular risk posed by technology. Her argument is that historical and social changes have led to the dominance of values that advocate human goodness, purity and equality (secularism) (Douglas 1969, 1975, 1992). The threats to these values are conspiracy and worldliness. These threats appear in the form of hidden scientific and technological contamination. These underlying social values have determined Western societies' focus in their selection of risk and the establishing of blame. This explains how in the space of fifteen to twenty years technology has changed from being regarded as a source of safety to a source of risk (Douglas and Wildavsky 1982).

The dissatisfaction with formal scientific medicine has had a number of consequences. It has awakened an interest in the use of diverse traditional and alternative medicine. 'In an unpredictable, dangerous, anxiety ridden world, people flock to the marketplace to purchase magical goods and services' (Kassell 2005: 47). There is, for example, a return to ancient ideas and practices such as neo-Paganism and New Age philosophies that claim continuities with the past (Heelas 1996). Increased disposable income and consumer philosophy have aided the move to high trends in the utilisation of alternative healthcare (see Eisenberg et al. 2001; McQuaide 2005). Alternative medicine is increasingly big business in Britain (and the U.S.) and is increasingly subject to pressures to commoditise. In this 'New Age' it is the middle and upper-middle classes who are seen to take most advantage of complementary and alternative medicine (CAM) services, and in this light it may now be seen as a form of health inequality (McQuaide 2005).

In Britain there is currently a debate around whether the British Medical Association (BMA) should fund alternative medicine. Officially, and historically, formal medicine has displayed an aggressively dismissive attitude to CAM on the grounds that it is not scientific (see BMA 1986), although concessions were made to particular CAM practices in subsequent reports (BMA 1993; House of Lords 2000). In addition, we know that primary-care physicians do refer patients to alternative treatments (see Moore, Chapter 5, this volume). Also, younger doctors in Britain appear to be adopting more favourable attitudes towards alternative therapies (McQuaide 2005: 289). While this may not suggest evidence of a culture shift it might be evidence of a move toward openness within formal medicine, and a recognition that alternative treatments are not diminishing in popularity. It recognises multiple or parallel dynamics exist and undermines the idea that a singular health system dominates.

Yet, as Sharma (1991) suggests, orthodox medicine requires that alternative medicine be subjected to scientific testing. It insists that efficacy can be tested by standardised double blind trials. Sharma argues that few systems for alternative treatment rely solely on the ingestion of drugs or other substances, insisting that if there is little 'objective' evidence that alternative medicine works better than orthodox medicine, there is at least evidence that it has many satisfied clients.

The likely reason that Western medicine publicly continues to reject, dismiss or ignore CAM lies in the fear that the formal sanctioning of alternative practices will have major economic, political and social consequences that will undermine the role and position of medical practitioners. Recognition of alternative medicine would mean, in part, recognition of failures in the practice of biomedicine. For example, Sharma suggests that alternative medicine is generally found to be a response to one or more of those chronic conditions for which modern medicine offers only limited relief. It is partly a dissatisfaction with conventional medicine, and/or the physician–patient relationship, that 'drives' the patient to the unorthodox healer (Sharma 1991). So even if the actual specific health benefits are nebulous or illusory, the secondary aspects of such a belief system benefit the community at large. We should also consider the magical and illusory within formal biomedicine.[9]

The prominent sociologist Pierre Bourdieu recognised the false dichotomy between the supernatural/traditional/primitive and the rational/modern/civilised. For Bourdieu, the question is about the 'universe of practice' versus 'the universe of academic discourse' (Bowie 2006: 227). In other words, there appears to be, as Bowie underlines, a system of logic and fuzzy logic where systems contradict each other, but interact and play simultaneously. This is because health and medicine are such a serious concern that they require a pragmatic understanding that extends beyond scientific rationalism and offer the use of multiple medical resources. Bowie illustrates how Bourdieu bridges the apparent paradox and contradictions of spiritual and scientific belief and the position held, for example, by fundamentalist Christian scientists. While the philosophies behind religion and science (and paradigms that underpin them) may appear to conflict, in reality they pragmatically co-exist and are interdependent both in advanced and traditional societies. In short, religiosity, spirituality, magic and rationality are not mutually exclusive: 'There is a scientific way of thinking that tests hypotheses against everyday reality and experience, essential to technical advances, and a more 'mystical' or non-logical mode of thought that works via metaphor and analogy to make sense of the complexity of human existence. In practice these may not be distinguishable from one another, or may both come into play in the same situation' (ibid.: 225–26).

The scientific world is underpinned with the search for certainties. Propositions are tested or disproved through empirical observations. What is produced is evidence-based logic which now informs health and medical (evidence-based) practice. This is the scripture of the medical school and the mantra of the nursing faculty. It provides a certain type of knowledge and understanding, but paradoxically, it limits the boundary of our understanding by virtue of its mechanistic rubric – a rational scientific framework. That which cannot be easily or readily explained is often cast out as conjecture, myth and bunkum.

Thus, 'neo-positive philosophies of science accept scientific theory unproblematically as representing a reality that is "out there"' (Stepnisky 2007: 189–90). Yet, awkward questions remain and are unanswered. For example, important ontological and epistemological questions arise, to summon Kant and the idea of what counts as real. Does only the empirically observable count as real, or are there other more complex realities that need to be considered? Such philosophical questions, which we merely pose here, lead us to a consideration of what has been described as the complexity turn (Blaikie 2007).

Bhaskar (2002) reminds us that social ontology serves to conceptualise social reality in certain terms, thus identifying what there is to be explained. This also rules out other possible explanations (Archer 1995). While Bhaskar points up the implication of this, in a consideration of the ontology of social class – itself a contested concept (see Pakulski and Watters 1996) – Scambler and Higgs point to the 'real' consequences that may lie beyond our understanding of the immediate and observed (Scambler and Higgs 1999). Bhaskar's position of critical realism (Bhaskar 2002) and the later 'complexity turn' discussed by Blaikie (2007) goes some way to address the idea that reality exists independently of and beyond our experiences and knowledge, and we briefly acknowledge these contributions (see also Archer et al. 1998).

Conclusion

In highlighting the foundations of health beliefs and healthcare systems, we have begun to tease out the importance of the role of cosmology, religion and magic in the formation of folk beliefs and practices in Britain and Ireland. In so doing, we have also illuminated the role of science and the complex and evolving interface between science, superstition, religion and magic in the era of modernity. As we have discussed in this chapter, folk healing refers to multiple and culturally varied health belief systems that rest not on universal laws but on a wide spectrum of specific 'organic' healing beliefs, traditions and practices. An all-encompassing definition of folk healing or folk medicine is problematic, not least due to the diversity of past and currently existing folk-healing practices and beliefs.

A key theme of the chapter that we can extrapolate here is the relationship –sometimes paradoxical, always problematic – between folk medicine and biomedicine; between scientific, rational explanations and spiritual or folk beliefs. Without wishing to add to familiar dichotomies, our discussion has clearly cast a spotlight over the socio-historical and contemporary tensions that such dichotomies give rise to. This complex situation is equally obviated by our understanding of the peculiar modernity (or modernities) from which such tensions emerge. Whether the advent of late-modernity or new modernities will increasingly problematise this relationship is a key question that should be posed by future studies of both formal medicine and folk healing.

Notes

1. For the most part the nomenclature and terminology is nebulous and cumbersome. Folk medicine has been variously described as ethnomedicine, indigenous medicine, or healing separate and within a localised and locally defined set of beliefs and practices. It has also been described as complementary medicine, which assumes recognition of the superior status and position of Western biomedicine.
2. Cosmology refers to the nature of the universe and the place of people within it. Cosmogony refers to myths, legends and stories that seek to explain the origin of the universe and people within it.
3. Lambek provides detailed objections to Tylor's assertions and the evolutionary ideas on which they were based (Lambek 2002).
4. 'Quack' is derived from the sixteenth-century Dutch word *Quacksalver*, meaning one who quacks like a duck and boasts about the virtues of his ointments (Gevitz 1988).
5. Chapter 3 (this volume) provides a discussion of this in the Irish historical context.
6. Wallis and Morley point to the established recognition of 'Germ Theory' as a crucial component of this legitimacy and consensus amongst physicians (Wallis and Morley 1976: 13).
7. Source: *Channel 4 News*, 3 September 2007.

8. The debate is compounded further by parallel and ongoing debates exploring 'reflexive modernity' (Giddens 1991; Beck 1992; Beck, Giddens and Lasch 1994) or 'second modernity' (Beck and Lau 2005; Beck 2006). Such theories have examined how present socio-cultural change is representative of a new stage of modernity, and not a distinct era.
9. A recent BBC documentary on the evidence for alternative medicine, broadcast in 2005, discussed a major trial in the U.S.A. that examined the placebo effects of surgery for arthritis of the knee. While some patients had a normal operation performed on their knee, others had their skin incised and then sewn up again. Both groups had the same positive outcomes from the procedures. The effect shows that it may be possible to harness the positive powers from a person's mind and body to heal itself.

References

Ackerknect, E. 1946. 'Natural Diseases and Rational Treatment in Primitive Medicine', *Bulletin of the History of Medicine* 19: 467–97.

Andreski, S. 1980. 'The Syphilitic Shock: Puritanism, Capitalism and the Medical Factor', *Encounter* 55(4): 76–81.

Archer, M. 1995. *Realist Social Theory: The Morphogenetic Approach*. Cambridge: Cambridge University Press.

Archer, M., R. Bhaskar, A. Collier, T. Lawson and A. Norrie (eds). 1998. *Critical Realism: Essential Readings*. London: Routledge.

Bakx, K. 1991. 'The Eclipse of Folk Medicine in Western Society', *Sociology of Health and Illness* 13(1): 20–38.

Ballance, L. 2002. 'Integrating CAM Into a Group Practice: The Experience of The Permanente Medical Group in Northern California', *The Permanente Journal, Complementary and Alternative Medicine* 6(4): 54–56 .

Barrett R., R. Moore and A. Staines. 2007. 'Blood Transfusion in Ireland: Perceptions of Risk, a Question of Trust', *Health, Risk and Society* 9(4): 375–88.

Bauman, Z. 1995. *Life in Fragments*. Oxford: Blackwell.

Beck, U. 1992. *Risk Society: Towards a New Modernity*. London: Sage.

______. 2006. 'Risky Business', *Guardian*, 11 February.

Beck, U., A. Giddens and S Lasch. 1994. *Reflexive Modernization: Politics, Tradition and Aesthetics in the Modern Social Order*. Cambridge: Polity Press.

Beck, U. and C. Lau, C. 2005. Second Modernity as a Research Agenda: Theoretical and Empirical Explorations in the 'Meta-change' of Modern Society. *British Journal of Sociology* 56(4): 525–57.

Bendix, R. 1966. *Max Weber: An Intellectual Portrait*. London: Methuen.

Benko, S. 1993. *Virgin Goddess: Studies in the Pagan and Christian Roots of Mariology*. Leiden: Brill.

Bhaskar, R. 2002. *Reflections On Meta-Reality: A Philosophy for the Present*. London: Sage

Blackman, W. 1918. 'The Rosary in Magic and Religion', *Folklore* 29(4): 255–80.

Blaikie, N. 2007. *Approaches to Social Inquiry*, 2nd edn. Cambridge: Polity.

Bowie, F. 2006. *The Anthropology of Religion: An Introduction*, 2nd edn. Oxford: Blackwell.

BMA. 1986. 'Alternative Therapy'. London: British Medical Association.

______. 1993. *Complementary Medicine: New Approaches to Good Practice*. Oxford: Oxford University Press.

Broca, P. 1876. 'Sur l'âge des sujets à la trépanation chirurgicale néolithique', *Bulletin* de la Société d'*Anthropologie* de Paris,. Sér 2, 11: 572.

Bynum, W.F. and R. Porter (eds). 1987. *Medical Fringe and Medical Orthodoxy, 1750–1850*. London: Croom Helm.

Cant, S. and U. Sharma. 1999. *A New Medical Pluralism? Alternative Medicine, Doctors, and the State*. London: UCL Press.

Clark, S. 1997. *Thinking with Demons: The Idea of Witchcraft in Early Modern Europe*. Oxford: Oxford University Press.

Coe, R.M. 1997. 'The Magic of Science and the Science of Magic: An Essay on the Process of Healing', *Journal of Health and Social Behavior* 38: 1–8.

Douglas, M. 1969. *Purity and Danger: An Analysis of Concepts of Pollution and Taboo*. London: Routledge and Kegan Paul.

______. 1975. *Implicit Meanings: Essays in Anthropology*. London: Routledge.

______. 1992. *Risk and Blame: Essays in Cultural Theory*. London: Routledge.

Douglas, M. and A. Wildavsky. 1982. *Risk and Culture*. Berkeley: University of California Press.

Durkheim, E. 1976[1915]. *Elementary Forms of Religious Life*. London: Allen and Unwin.

Easthope, G. 1986. *Healers and Alternative Medicine: A Sociological Examination*. Aldershot: Gower Publishing.

Ehrenreich, B. and D. English. 1972. *Witches, Midwives and Nurses: A History of Women Healers*. London: Feminist Press, Glass Mountain Pamphlets.

Ehrenwald, J. 1956. *From Medicine Man to Freud*. New York: Dell Publishing Company.

Eisenberg, D.M., T. Kaptchuk, C. Laine and F. Davidoff. 2001. 'Complementary and Alternative Medicine: An Annals Series', *Annals of Internal Medicine* 135(3): 208.

Estes, L. 1983. 'The Medical Origins of the European Witch Crazes: A Hypothesis', *Journal of Social History* 17(2): 271–84.

Evans-Pritchard, E.E. 1937. *Witchcraft, Oracles, and Magic among the Azande*. London: Oxford University Press.

Finger S and H Fernando 2001. 'E. George Squier and the Discovery of Cranial Trepanation: A Landmark in the History of Surgery and Ancient Medicine', Journal of the History of Medicine and Allied Sciences 56(4) 353–81.

Frankenberg, R. 1980. 'Medical Anthropology and Development: A Theoretical Perspective', *Social Science and Medicine* 148: 197–207.

Frazer, J.G. 1911. *The Golden Bough*. London: Macmillan.

Friedman, D. 1981. 'Anatomy of Ambiguous Folk Medicine', in, T. Vaskilampi and C. MacCormack (eds), *Folk Medicine and Health Culture: The Role of Folk Medicine in Modern Health Care*. Kuopio: Department of Community Health, University of Kuopio.

Gevitz, N. 1988. 'Three Perspectives on Unorthodox Medicine', in N. Gevitz (ed.) *Other Healers: Unorthodox Medicine in America*. Baltimore, MD: John Hopkins University Press.

Giddens, A. 1990 . *The Consequences of Modernity*. Cambridge: Polity Press.

———. 1991. *Modernity and Self Identity*. Cambridge: Polity Press.

Good, B.J. 1994. *Medicine, Rationality and Experience: An Anthropological Perspective*. Cambridge: Cambridge University Press.

Graham, J. 1985. 'Folk Medicine and Intracultural Diversity among West Texas Mexican Americans', *Western Folklore* 4(3): 168–93.

Hamilton, M. 2005. *The Sociology of Religion: Theoretical and Comparative Perspectives*, 2nd edn. London: Routledge.

Hardey, M. 1999. '"Doctor in the House": The Internet as a Source of Lay Health Knowledge and the Challenge to Expertise', *Sociology of Health and Illness* 21(6): 820–36.

Harrison, J.F.C. 1987. 'Early Victorian Radicals and the Medical Fringe', in W.F. Bynum and R. Porter (eds), *Medical Fringe and Medical Orthodoxy, 1750–1850*. London: Croom Helm.

Heelas, P. 1996. *The New Age Movement: Religion, Culture and Society in the Age of Postmodernity*. Oxford: Blackwell.

Hesse, B.W., D. Nelson, G. Kreps, R. Croyle, N. Arora, B. Rimer and K. Viswanath. 2005. 'Trust and Sources of Health Information', *Archives of Internal Medicine* 165: 2618–24.

House of Lords. 2000. 'Complementary and Alternative Medicine', report of the Select Committee on Science and Technology. HL Paper 123. London: HMSO.

Kaptchuk, T. and M. Croucher. 1987. *The Healing Arts: A Journey through the Faces of Medicine*. New York: Summit Books.

Kaptchut, T. and D. Eisenberg. 2001. 'Varieties of Healing. A Taxonomy of Unconventional Healing Practice', *Annals of Internal Medicine* 135(3): 196–204.

Kassell, L. 2005a. 'The Economy of Magic in Early Modern England', in M. Pelling and S. Mandelbrot (eds), *The Practice of Reform in Health, Medicine and Science, 1500–2000: Essays for Charles Webster*. Aldershot: Ashgate.

______. 2005b. *Medicine and Magic in Elizabethan London*. Oxford: Clarendon Press.

______. 2006. '"All Was this Land Full Fill'd of Faerie", or Magic and the Past in Early Modern England', *Journal of the History of Ideas* 67(1): 107–22.

Kelleher, D., J. Gabe and G. Williams. 1994. 'Understanding Medical Dominance in the Modern World', in J. Gabe, D. Kelleher and G. Williams (eds), *Challenging Medicine*. London: Routledge.

LaFontaine, J. 1998. *Speak of the Devil: Tales of Satanic Abuse in Contemporary England*. Cambridge: Cambridge University Press.

Lambek, M. 2002. *A Reader in the Anthropology of Religion*. Oxford: Blackwell.

Lane, J. 2001. *A Social History of Medicine*. London: Routledge.

Lawrence, C. 1994. *Medicine in the Making of Modern Britain, 1700–1920*. London: Routledge.

Leslie, C. (ed.) 1977. *Asian Medical Systems: A Comparative Study*. Berkeley: University of California Press.

Lindquist, G. 2005. *Conjuring Hope: Healing and Magic in Contemporary Russia*. Oxford: Berghahn.

Lupton, D. 1994. *Medicine as Culture: Illness, Disease and the Body in Western Societies*. London: Sage.

McGuire, M. and D. Kantor. 1987. 'Belief Systems and Illness Experiences: The Case of Non-medical Healing Groups', *Research in the Sociology of Health Care* 6: 221–48.

McQuaide, M. 2005. 'The Rise of Alternative Health Care: A Sociological Account', *Social Theory and Health* 3(4): 286–301.

Malinowski, B. 1974[1948] *Magic, Science and Religion, and Other Essays*. London: Souvenir Press.

Mathews, F. 1994. *The Ecological Self*. London: Routledge.

Mauss, M. and H. Hubert. 1972[1902]. *A General Theory of Magic*. London: Routledge and Kegan Paul.

Neve, M. 1987. 'Orthodoxy and Fringe: Medicine in Late Georgian Bristol', in W.F. Bynum and R. Porter (eds), *Medical Fringe and Medical Orthodoxy, 1750–1850*. London: Croom Helm.

Pakulski, J. and M. Watters. 1996. *The Death of Class*. London: Sage.

Pels, P. 2003. 'Introduction: Magic and Modernity', in B. Meyer and P. Pels (eds), *Magic and Modernity*. Stanford, CA: Stanford University Press.

Porter, R. 1993. *Disease, Medicine and Society in England, 1550–1860*. London: Macmillan.

———. 1998 *The Greatest Benefit to Mankind: A Medical History of Humanity*. London: Harper Collins.

Quave, C.L. and A. Pieroni. 2005. 'Ritual Healing in Arbereshe Albanian and Italian Communities of Lucania, Southern Italy', *Journal of Folklore Research* 42(1): 57–97.

Ramsey, M. 1999. 'Alternative Medicine in Modern France', *Historical Medicine* 43: 286–322.

Rivers, W.H.R. 2001[1924]. *Medicine, Magic and Religion*. London: Routledge.

Rorty, R. 1987. 'Pragmatism and Philosophy', in K. Baynes, J. Bothman, and T. McCarthy (eds), *After Philosophy*. Cambridge, MA: MIT Press.

———. 1989. *Contingency, Irony and Solidarity*. Cambridge: Cambridge University Press.

Saks, M. 1991. 'Power, Politics and Alternative Medicine', *Talking Politics* 3(2): 68–72.

———. 1994. 'The Alternatives to Medicine', in J. Gabe, D. Kelleher and G. Williams (eds), *Challenging Medicine*. London: Routledge.

———. 1998. 'Medicine and Complementary Medicine: Challenge and Change', in G. Scambler and P. Higgs (eds), *Modernity, Medicine and Health: Medical Sociology Towards 2000*. London: Routledge.

———. 2001. 'Alternative Medicine and the Health Care Division of Labour: Present Trends and Future Prospects', *Current Sociology* 49(3): 119–34.

Saks, M. (ed.) 1992. *Alternative Medicine in Britain*. Oxford: Clarendon Press.

Salmon, J.W. 1984. 'Introduction', in J.W. Salmon (ed.) *Alternative Medicines. Popular and Policy Perspectives*. London: Tavistock.

Sanders, A. 1995. *A Deed without a Name: The Witch in Society and History* Oxford: Berg.

Scambler, G. and P. Higgs. 1999. 'Stratification, Class and Health: Class Relations and Health Inequalities in High Modernity', *Sociology* 33(2) 275–96.

Sharma, U. 1991. 'Using "Alternative Medicine", *Health Visitor* 64(2): 50–51.

Smart, B. 1993. *Postmodernity*. London: Routledge.

Stacey, M. 1988. *The Sociology of Health and Healing*. London: Routledge.

Stepnisky, J. 2007. 'The Biomedical Self: Hermeneutics Considerations', *Social Theory and Health* 5(3): 187–207.

Stringer, M. 1999. 'Rethinking Animism: Thoughts from the Infancy of Our Discipline', *Journal of the Royal Anthropological Institute* 5(4): 541–55.

Tambiah, S.J. 1990. *Magic, Science, Religion, and the Scope of Rationality*. Cambridge: Cambridge University Press,

Thomas, K. 1973. *Religion and the Decline of Magic*. London: Penguin.

———. 1975. 'An Anthropology of Religion and Magic, II', *Journal of Interdisciplinary History* l6(1): 99–109.

Thompson, K. 1992. 'Social Pluralism and Postmodernity', in S. Hall, D. Held and T. McGrew (eds), *Modernity and its Futures*. Cambridge: Polity Press.

Turner, B. 1991 *Religion and Social Theory*. London: Sage.

______. 2000. The History of the Changing Concepts of Health and Illness: Outline of a General Model of Illness Categories, in G. Albrecht, R. Fitzpatrick and S. Scrimshaw (eds), *The Handbook of Social Studies in Health and Medicine*. London: Sage.

Tylor E.B. 1958[1871] *Primitive Culture*. London: John Murray.

Ulett, G. 1992. *Beyond Yin and Yang. How Acupuncture Really Works*. St Louis, MO: Warren Green Inc.

Van Gennep, A. 1937. *Manuel de foklore française contemporain*. Paris. Picard.

Wallis, R. and P. Morley. (eds). 1976. *Marginal Medicine*. London: Peter Owen.

Whiteford, L. and L. LaCivita Nixon. 2000. Comparative Health Systems: Emerging Convergences and Globalisation, in G. Albrecht, R. Fitzpatrick and S. Scrimshaw (eds), *The Handbook of Social Studies in Health and Medicine*. London: Sage.

Chapter 3

The Medical Marketplace and Medical Tradition in Nineteenth-century Ireland

Catherine Cox

In 1895, the charred body of Bridget Cleary, a 26-year-old woman, was found in a shallow grave in County Tipperary in Ireland. The immediate events that culminated in her death appeared to originate in a cold she caught which necessitated bed rest. As her illness proved resilient to all forms of medical intervention, her husband Michael Cleary became convinced, or was persuaded, that the fairies had abducted his real wife.[1] In his attempts to establish the true identity of the sick woman he burned his wife to death. This gruesome story and the associated criminal proceedings have been ascribed multiple meanings. Among other factors, Bourke has emphasised that, as a dressmaker, Bridget was a 'modern woman', and the combined income of the couple 'placed them far ahead of most rural working people' (Bourke 1999: 45). She also draws attention to the fraught political climate of late nineteenth-century Ireland and identifies nationalists' fears that the 'uncivilised' events surrounding the death of Bridget Cleary in 1895 would undermine their demands for home rule and impugn their capacity for self-government (Bourke 1995; 1999).

At the heart of this incident is, of course, patient and familial behaviour in response to illness. During the early attempts to cure Bridget, her family sought the assistance of the local dispensary doctor, William Crean. However, there was a four-day delay before Crean attended the Cleary home for the first time. He left instructions that the patient be given certain medicines but subsequently stated that he did not know if they were administered. Bridget did not improve and in frustration Michael discarded the medicine prescribed by Crean and sought out the ministrations of the local 'fairy' doctor. On the face of it, two medical systems are set up in conflict: biomedicine and its mechanisms of delivery are rejected as ineffectual in favour of the familiar and traditional. On the other hand, while the incident appears to contribute to the 'debunking' of Keith Thomas's theory of the 'disenchantment of the world', it also re-enforces the argument that by the end of the nineteenth century patients had not 'developed an exclusive preference for a particular therapy' (Gijswijt-Hofstra, Marland and de Waardt 1997: 5).

The programme of research, of which this chapter is an early and tentative product, will endeavour to explore some of the questions prompted by these and similar events (Hoff and Yeates 2000; Prior 2006). Ultimately, the project endeavours not only to identify the various medical options available in late eighteenth- and nineteenth-century Irish society, but also to interrogate the extent to which they represented conflicting medical systems, as they are often portrayed. Crucially, the overall project intends to come to a better understanding of patient behaviour. As Bivins (2007: 3) has shown, by the early nineteenth century, patients readily accessed and participated in a variety of medical processes and innovations. In considering patients' choice of practitioner, emphasis has been placed upon the operation of the medical marketplace – the patients' willingness to shop around – and the efficacy and cost of treatment (Porter 2000: 42–43, 115–30). However, the historian must be wary of adopting an exclusively functionalist interpretation. In the case of Bridget Cleary, it is unclear whether bioscience per se was rejected due to its failure to cure Bridget or if its agent of delivery, the dispensary doctor, was perceived as problematic. Crean's delay in visiting the household and his reputation for drunkenness appear to have provoked Michael Cleary's consultation of the fairy doctor as much as the failure to cure Bridget. The 'ethical' character of the practitioner could also influence patient choice (McKay 2005).

Before an interrogation of patient behaviour can be engaged upon, the available medical repertoire, and the interactions between all practitioners, must also be assessed. This chapter will explore the historic relationship between 'folk', 'alternative' and 'regular' medical approaches to disease, illness and treatment and suggest that the characterisation of it as an exclusively hostile dichotomy is a simplification. Undoubtedly, the late eighteenth and nineteenth centuries witnessed the broadening of access to regular medical provision in Ireland. This took the form of the expansion and consolidation of regular practitioners, including dispensary doctors, the extension of institutional provision, and associated employment opportunities. However, the piecemeal nature of this process did not lead to the displacement of older existing practices of medical healing and the concomitant denigration of these practices. As Bradley has indicated, terms such as 'heterodox' and 'folk' place these practices 'outside the realms of the dominant form of medicine as "alternative", "fringe" and "marginal"' (Bradley 2002: 19). The divisions between 'regular', 'quack' and 'folk', often delineated by regular practitioners, are arguably social constructions, and may not have been shared by patients (Porter 1992: 8; Ernst 2002: 1–18; Peeters 2008). The criticisms inherent in the labelling of practitioners would not have had relevance to the patients themselves as they shopped around in the medical marketplace.[2] Among patients in Ireland, heterodox practices occupied a central position in medical provision and their continued existence encouraged 'orthodox' practitioners to incorporate aspects of their therapeutics. In their characterisations of various healing practices and their respective knowledge claims, 'regular' practitioners' attitudes were shaped by a vast range of criteria, and the vying influences of antiquarianism, scientific rationality and cultural revivalism are all identifiable. While rejecting some heterodox practices, contributors to medical and literary publications appear to legitimise others through the deployment of scientific rationality contributing to the blurring of boundaries between orthodoxy and heterodoxy.

Fundamentally, attitudes towards heterodox practitioners were influenced by levels of competition in the medical marketplace. An insight into the distribution of medical practitioners and regulatory legislation and bodies is a necessary starting point for any assessment of patient choice and the interfaces between individuals engaged in medicine as an occupation (Pelling and Webster 1979). Historians of medicine in Ireland have not fully mapped the distribution of medical practitioners as part of an overall assessment of the level of 'overstocking' in the Irish medical marketplace. Geary (2004: 134) and Ó Gráda (1994: 187) have interrogated the distribution of regular practitioners during the period of the Great Famine. Geary supplements the material in the census returns with Henry Croly's medical directories of 1843 and 1846 (Geary 2004: 134). Thus, while studies have revealed something of the institutions and personalities of Irish medical history, little is known about practitioners' 'number, diversity, distribution and availability' (Digby 2002: 11).[3]

Regulation and the Medical Marketplace

By 1900 in Ireland, as elsewhere, the structure of regular practice and its attendant regulatory bodies had been significantly renegotiated (Digby 2002: 2). Historically, the Royal College of Physicians of Ireland and the Royal College of Surgeons of Ireland, often engaged in lively rivalry with one another, were the dominant interest groups and regulatory bodies for surgeons and physicians prior to the passage of the 1858 Medical Act (21 and 22 Vict. c.90, 2 August 1858). The Royal College of Physicians was granted its first charter by Charles II in 1667 and was, theoretically, responsible for licensing 'graduates in physic' (Fleetwood 1983: 32–36). Surgeons were formally separated from the Company of Barber Surgeons in 1784 when the Royal College of Surgeons was granted a charter by George III (ibid.: 70–71). These two bodies, in conjunction with the Apothecaries' Hall, were legislatively responsible for the regulation of medical practice in Ireland, although the effectiveness and indeed the appetite for enforcement is debateable. The campaign for the reform of the regulation and structure of medical practice was debated with vitriol in Britain and culminated in the 1858 Medical Act.[4] The Act and its attendant limitations, was eventually introduced to Ireland. According to Fleetwood, the Act required the Royal College of Surgeons to 'combine with a licensing body competent to grant medical degrees or diplomas' (ibid.: 75). To secure this, they reached an arrangement with the Royal College of Physicians. The Act appeared to place the apothecaries in an anomalous position. From the early eighteenth century, apothecaries were required to register with the Royal College of Physicians. However, during the ensuing decades apothecaries sought greater autonomy from physicians as evidenced by the establishment of Apothecaries' Hall under legislation passed in 1791 (31 Geo. III 1791). The 1791 Act also conferred on them a 'monopoly on the importation and distribution of drugs into Ireland' (ibid.: 88). The Apothecaries' Hall performed a limited regulatory function granting certificates to apprentices, assistants and journeymen, and to apothecary shops. Between 1791 and 1829 the Hall issued 5,000 certificates to qualified apprentices, 463 to assistants and journeymen, and 1,289 to apothecaries seeking to establish themselves in business.[5] Offences under the terms of the Act included setting up shop without a licence, appointing uncertified apprentices or assistants, and selling arsenic. Between 1791 and 1829 there were 194 successful cases brought against individuals throughout Ireland who had established apothecary shops without licences.[6] Despite the apparent monopoly, the apothecaries echoed the demands of their English counterparts for more restrictive measures against 'quacks', but they were not successful.[7] Even the disappointing 1815 Apothecaries Act was not extended to Ireland and, consequently, apothecaries continued to be regulated by the 1791 Act. While the 1858 Medical Act recognised the Apothecaries' Hall as a licensing body (ibid.: 81–94), Dublin medical circles expressed some dissatisfaction at the apothecaries' position under its terms and engaged in a campaign highlighting its defects in the *Dublin Medical Press*.[8]

Regular practitioners' attitudes towards heterodox practice were articulated within the dynamics of the medical marketplace. Medical historians of England have emphasised the tensions between various practitioners operating in an overstocked medical marketplace and have identified campaigns for professional status as central to the hostility displayed towards different groups. Irvine Loudon's exploration of regular practitioners' attitudes towards emerging druggists has stressed the economic context of the debate and the threat that druggists posed to the trade of the apothecaries (Loudon 1987). There was similar hostility displayed towards other groups – hydropathists, homeopaths and doctresses to name a few – who had identified a niche area in the market for their wares and specialisms (Cooter 1988). While Ireland exhibits some similar characteristics, the social, economic and cultural conditions in which Irish practitioners worked differed significantly. The extent to which a medical marketplace predicated on the presence of expanding consumerism could be sustained in Ireland is as yet a matter of debate. Outside Dublin,[9] industrialisation was confined mainly to the north-east while the rest of Ireland remained predominantly, though not exclusively, rural. For much of the nineteenth century, the country experienced significant economic hardships. While the Great Famine (1845–1850) dominates Irish historiography, there were other periods of extreme distress both prior to and following the Great Famine.[10] There were also periods of economic boom, such as occurred in the late 1870s, which had a significant impact upon the wealth of the country and facilitated the emergence of medical institutions and practitioners (Ó Gráda 1994: 236–54).

Urbanisation was piecemeal, and outside the larger cities many of the provincial towns shared the general pattern of emigration and population decline. Consequently in a predominately rural country, the workforce largely comprised agricultural labourers. There was, however, an expansion of a middle class by the late nineteenth century (Vaughan 1989: 740). The demographic profile of the country, while not unique, differed from general European trends (Daly 2006: 3–17). The population growth of the 1700s had slowed by the beginning of the nineteenth century and during the period following the Great Famine the population declined significantly due to the combined impact of the death rate during the Great Famine, emigration and delayed births (Guinnane 1999). Regular practitioners did not escape these trends. According to the census returns, by 1851, the number of physicians and surgeons in Ireland had declined by 14.4 per cent. Emigration was a constant feature of nineteenth-century Irish life, both before and after the Great Famine and regular medical practitioners formed part of the post-famine exodus (Jones 2006). Ireland was also mixed culturally, denominationally and linguistically. By 1871, 'just over three-quarters of the population' were Catholics; 12 per cent were members of the Church of Ireland and a further 9 per cent were Presbyterians (Vaughan 1989: 738–39). It is estimated that only 34 per cent of doctors were Catholic in 1870 (ibid.: 741). The Irish language, while in decline, was still spoken mainly on the western seaboard, including counties Mayo, Donegal and Cork, at the end of the nineteenth century.

This environment undoubtedly presented the Irish medical practitioner with a variety of opportunities and hindrances when 'making a medical living'. To assess the level of competition and access in different contexts, the distribution of medical practitioners in seven counties in Ireland (Dublin, Cork, Kilkenny, Carlow, Donegal, Kerry and Mayo) has been mapped. The counties incorporate regions exhibiting significant linguistic distance between patient and practitioner, varying urban and rural contrasts, and proximity to larger cities. The counties experienced the expansion of communication networks at different stages while the topography of medical institutional development varied considerably. The seven counties chosen facilitate an assessment of several important questions in various socio-economic contexts. At this early stage of the project, the selection of counties rather than towns or cities as the unit of analysis attempts to acknowledge the fluidity of the boundaries between urbanized centres and rural hinterlands in the consideration of medical provision and networks (Mortimer 2007: 72).

Sources

The sources interrogated in the assessment of the distribution of practitioners include the Irish medical directories – both pre and post the 1858 Medical Act – various eighteenth- and nineteenth-century city and county trade directories, and university rolls containing details of student entrants. These have been supplemented by numerous parliamentary reports, including censuses, published returns and accounts of the Poor Law commissioners, the lunacy inspectorates, the Apothecaries' Hall, and the committees established to inquire into the condition of the poor in Ireland and the medical charities. In the completed project, it is intended to deploy Margaret Pelling's definition of a medical practitioner (Pelling and Webster 1979), that is someone who is engaged in medicine as an occupation rather than a profession (Digby 2002: 26) as the criteria of inclusion.[11] Consequently, returns for dentists, chemists, druggists, opticians and truss-makers, in addition to physicians, surgeons and apothecaries will be included in the analysis. This incorporates self-styled medical practitioners in addition to fellows, members and licentiates of the different colleges. This will facilitate a thorough consideration of the variety of options available to the patient in eighteenth- and nineteenth-century Ireland. However, at this early stage the analysis of the distribution of practitioners has been limited to surgeons, physicians and apothecaries. The surgeons and physicians were listed in the respective medical directories of the nineteenth century. The returns for the apothecaries have been gleaned from trade directories, and although the majority claimed to be licentiates of the Apothecaries' Hall, a small number of self-styled practitioners were undoubtedly present.

As Digby has noted in her analysis of practitioners in England and Wales, the source material for this type of study is problematic (Digby 2002: 5–11). In the case of Ireland, there are even greater difficulties. The variety of sources from which to compile estimates of practising medical practitioners are less abundant (ibid.: 11). The main sources are the medical directories and registers. As Digby has shown, the discrepancies between the directories and the registers are not great. However, the medical directories present a variety of problems. The first reliable medical directory for Ireland alone was compiled by Henry Croly, a doctor and a licentiate of the Royal College of Surgeons from Queen's County (Geary 2004: 135). His directory appeared in 1843, followed by a 'condensed, cheap and improved' version in 1846. Croly intended the volumes to be used as a guide by his contemporary colleagues and it was compiled with their co-operation. Practitioners submitted their own returns, detailing their name, address and qualifications. The medical directory of 1852 has proved particularly problematic: data concerning qualifications did not correspond with the relevant university rolls, with inaccuracies in approximately 50 per cent of the directory entries. The entries for Dublin city and county are particularly ambiguous. A significant proportion of the physicians and surgeons did not return their details and consequently those who compiled the directory relied on data available elsewhere. In part, the failure of many physicians to make returns may have been a result of the Great Famine. Not only was the mortality rate high among doctors during the Great Famine (Froggatt 1989), they were also in a position to realise their assets and emigrate. Consequently, to minimise these problems where possible the medical directories have been supplemented by trade directories. They also provide details of practitioners styling themselves as apothecaries, druggists and so forth, who are not registered. While for some of the larger cities and towns, such as Dublin and Cork, trade directories were published relatively frequently, other regions are not as well served. The later medical directories are more reliable. The 1858 Medical Act ensured that the amount and accuracy of the statistical information improved, although some limitations remained (Digby 2002: 11).

There are also significant problems when using the census material The first census to exhibit any degree of reliability is 1841; there are serious limitations with the first three official censuses of 1813, 1821 and 1831. The first of these was 'never completed' while the enumerators employed on the 1821 and 1831 censuses were tax-collectors who collected information on families in districts by word of mouth which was subsequently recorded in notebooks. As Vaughan and Fitzpatrick have shown, the enumerators encountered various obstacles: there was 'uncertainty concerning county boundaries', 'local people were often hostile', the 'collection of information did not take place simultaneously in all parts of the country' and 'enumerators believed they would be paid according to the numbers of people recorded.' Many of these problems were resolved following the establishment of the Census Commission and the first reliable census was published in 1841. In this instance the constabulary were used as enumerators and heads of households were supplied with forms on which to make returns (Vaughan and Fitzpatrick 1978: xii). Unfortunately, the manuscript returns of these censuses are not extant, leaving us dependent upon the published summaries. In addition, the 1851 census presents certain problems as it was compiled in the aftermath of the Great Famine. Therefore, while generally reliable, the nineteenth-century censuses do not allow the detailed cross-referencing of medical practitioners possible for England and Wales.

Distribution

Despite the various problems with the source material, the data does provide insight into patient access to medical provision. According to Digby there was a ratio of approximately one doctor to 950 patients in London in 1800, and by 1841 England 'was not far from this' (Digby 2002: 19). As a consequence of population growth, the ratio deteriorated until 1881, when a certain levelling out occurred. In Ireland, however, the doctor/patient ratio was at its best in 1861. In that year, Dublin city could boast one doctor to 478 patients while Cork had a ratio of one to 904. The provincial towns of Carlow and Kilkenny also fared reasonably well, although the numbers of regular practitioners was declining in Carlow town.[12] None of the urban areas examined have a ratio that is significantly worse than London. Nationally, the distribution of practitioners deteriorated after 1861.

This occurred in the context of a decline in the size of the Irish population, falling from around 6.5 million in 1851 to just under 4.5 million in 1901. There were significant regional differences in the rate of the decline and in the distribution of practitioners in the post-famine period. Dublin continued to be well served by regular practitioners: its lowest doctor/patient ratio was recorded in 1901 when there was one practitioner to 679 patients. The situation in Cork city was not as favourable, though it had improved by the end of the century. While urban access to regular practitioners was in line with England, none of the rural districts under consideration in this study even approximated the urban ratio. Unsurprisingly, County Mayo has the worst distribution: in 1861 there were 14,988 patients per doctor, improving to 3,557 in 1901. Excluding Dublin and Cork, most counties struggled to maintain a ratio of one regular practitioner to about 3200 patients. After 1871, the larger counties on the west coast, such as Kerry and Donegal, were not necessarily in a less favourable situation, and in 1891 both Kerry and Donegal were better served than Carlow and Kilkenny.[13] The numbers of practitioners recorded in the medical directories and other sources highlight the impact of the Great Famine not only on the doctor/patient ratio but also on administrative systems. There is a near uniform deterioration in the ratio for each city and county in the 1851 results. As discussed earlier, this was in part a result of the failure of practitioners to complete medical directory returns. However, the counties that exhibited the greatest deterioration in the doctor/patient ratio in 1852 – counties Donegal, Kerry and Mayo – correspond to the areas that were particularly hard hit during the Great Famine and by subsequent emigration.[14]

The distribution of regular practitioners was closely related to the development of institutional provisions. Unlike their English counterparts, practitioners in Georgian Ireland could not rely on the old Poor Law for opportunities, as the Elizabethan Poor Law legislation did not extend to Ireland. In eighteenth-century Ireland, a network of hospitals, infirmaries and dispensaries had been established often as a result of philanthropic and medical initiatives. These institutions depended upon subscriptions but these were seldom sufficient for their survival and consequently a large proportion of hospital and dispensary expansion in the later eighteenth and nineteenth centuries was the product of a high level of legislative provision for, and state support of, medical institutions. The establishment of county infirmaries and fever hospitals was encouraged by legislation passed in 1765 and 1807 respectively (O'Neill 1973). By 1846, county infirmaries were in operation in the majority of Irish counties (Geary 2004: 42). These institutions operated alongside the voluntary hospitals – specialists and general – and provided additional employment opportunities.

Amending legislation for the establishment of dispensaries, designed to provide free medicine and medical assistance to the poor, was enacted in 1805 (45 Geo. III c.111). Their development was hampered by funding difficulties, as they were dependent on local initiative, ensuring that their distribution was irregular (MacDonagh 1989: 208). Appointments to these institutions were highly competitive. The Royal College of Surgeons exercised a near 'monopoly over county infirmary appointments' from 1796 when legislation was enacted requiring all county infirmary surgeons to hold testimonial letters or a licence from the College (Geary 2004: 132–33). There was no legislative equivalent for practitioners appointed to dispensaries or fever hospitals who were not obliged to possess a particular medical qualification. As Geary has shown, medical appointments were often 'bought' and there was a 'religious imbalance' surrounding them which operated against Catholic practitioners (ibid.: 131).

The introduction of the Poor Law to Ireland in 1838 and the passage of the Medical Charities Act of 1851 provided new opportunities for regular practitioners. According to the 1851 Act, '723 dispensary districts were established with at least one dispensary in each district' (ibid.: 210). The expansion of the responsibilities of the Poor Law boards of guardians, obliging them to incorporate public health legislation and other initiatives, were also beneficial for regular practitioners seeking a stable source of income. For example, the 1858 smallpox vaccination act provided practitioners with a fee of £1 for every twenty cases (Brunton 1999: 149). Other opportunities emerged with the requirement to appoint regular medical attendants in prisons, factories, lunatic asylums, the military, the coastguard and insurance companies. The expansion of opportunities is reflected in the improvement in the doctor/patient ratio in both cities and counties after 1871.

This dependence on official posts ensured that the majority of nineteenth-century practitioners were largely supported by the state's purse. Ruth Barrington has suggested that by the later nineteenth century as much as half the registered medical practitioners in Ireland were employed as dispensary or workhouse medical officers (Barrington 2000: 16). The initial evidence from this study suggests that the figure was actually higher in some counties. By 1892 in County Donegal, approximately 65 per cent of the practitioners listed in the medical directory held state-funded appointments, and the figure was nearer 75 per cent in County Mayo. In Dublin, a post as a dispensary doctor facilitated surgeons who wished to maintain an unremunerated post at the more prestigious hospitals. At the beginning of his career, Lombe Athill, later Master of the Rotunda Hospital, remained as doctor to the Fleet Street dispensary in Dublin during the Great Famine. This allowed him to continue on the staff of a charitable institution (Athill 2007: 107–12).

Undoubtedly, the high dependence on such appointments ensured that the life of the surgeon or dispensary doctor in the larger rural districts was difficult. Dispensary doctors appointed after 1836 were obliged to live within 'five miles of the institution' (Geary 2004: 136), although there was some debate concerning this stipulation in the *Dublin Medical Press*.[15] This could result in a newly appointed doctor being obliged to rent basic accommodation on initial arrival in a dispensary district. In his recollections of a brief period spent as a dispensary doctor in Munster, Michael Joseph Malone recorded that his 'apartments were over a shop devoted to "public business," and as they had the advantage of being ceiled, a colony of rats took up their abode over them, under the shelter of the warm thatch' (Malone 1878: 73). Malone, writing for a mainly literary magazine (Clyde 2003), undoubtedly engaged in some hyperbole but his recollections have a ring of truth. He was listed in the Irish medical directory in the 1870s and was a member of the Royal Historical and Archaeological Association of Ireland. The residency stipulation could result in a prospective candidate for a position as a dispensary doctor being deemed ineligible for the post.[16] An appointment to a large dispensary district could also necessitate doctors travelling long distances to visit patients, much to their resentment. In 1879, Malone expressed some bitterness at the distances and conditions of travel the rural dispensary doctor was obliged to endure when compared to his urban counterpart:

> Practitioners, let me repeat, who have not had the actual experience of such work, and whom to a drive or walk of a few minutes will bring [him] to the bedside of ninety-five out of a hundred of their patients can hardly, from any mere description, form an adequate notion of the regions where good roads, intersect the district in all directions, and passable paths and byways lead up to every door, the doctor has at least one element of comfort in his cheerless drive in the silent hours of the night, often through pitiless rain and sleet. But there are localities in Ireland where roads do not run in nearly all directions, and where even travelling on horseback is quite impossible for a considerable portion – and that the worst portion – of the year. There the doctor ... has often to leave his bed to answer the sick-call on foot, over mountain and bog, depending on his way on the instincts rather than the vision of the guide who faithfully steers him through the rayless darkness of his destination. (Malone 1879: 383–84)

If Malone is to be believed, the ubiquitous rural doctors travelling on horseback present in contemporary caricatures were relatively absent from some parts of the Irish rural landscape. The columns of the *Dublin Medical Press* frequently attested to the alleged hardships and discomforts experienced by dispensary doctors.[17] It must be borne in mind that the editors of *Dublin Medical Press,* Arthur Jacob and Henry Maunsell, were staunch opponents of Whig philosophy and of the Medical Charities Bill (Kirkpatrick 1915: 1–13; Geary 2004: 162). The dispensary doctors were firmly convinced that their remuneration was not satisfactory compensation for these hardships and dispensary committees made repeated requests for salary increases on their behalf.[18] In 1858, the contributors to the *Dublin Medical Press* certainly felt they were underpaid. The salary of the Cork Union dispensary doctor was the subject of several articles published in the *Dublin Medical Press.*[19] However, by the late nineteenth century, the income derived from these posts was not insubstantial and certainly by 1872 the situation had improved. While there was variation, the average dispensary medical officer salary supplemented by smallpox vaccination fees had increased to over £100. The obligation to pay medical costs out of their salary obviously caused further resentment leading to one article in the *Dublin Medical Press* entitled 'Is Cod-Liver Oil a Medicine?'[20] However, by the 1880s, increasing numbers of practitioners held several appointments, possibly due to necessity, and their income could be supplemented further by private practice (see Malone 1878). Combined, these sources of income would place dispensary doctors' income on the border between the lower income scales of the middle classes and at the top of the small income categories devised by W.E. Vaughan (1989: 779). While these incomes may not have corresponded with the expectations of medical practitioners, it would suggest that by the late nineteenth century their complaints regarding poor pay may have been exaggerated.

Interfaces

Despite the expansion in opportunities and the possibility of a relatively secure income derived from state coffers, large sections of Ireland remained poorly served by regular practitioners in the nineteenth century. Patient access to dispensary doctors situated in larger districts in the provinces of Munster and Connaught could be problematic. Within this environment, there were ample opportunities for a variety of heterodox practitioners to maintain a secure patient base. The extant recollections and memoirs of dispensary doctors are sprinkled with references to a variety of 'folk'[21] practitioners and the medical journals attest to continued anxiety surrounding the presence of practitioners and practices delineated as 'quack' and 'charlatan' throughout the nineteenth century. While the towns and cities facilitated the emergence of increasing numbers of 'druggists and chemists', the local bone-setter and wise woman remained a consistent feature of Irish rural and urban society.

James Kelly (2005) has proposed that, similar to the English case, there was intense opposition to 'quackery' and similar practices in Ireland, particularly in Dublin in the eighteenth century. There was the predicable intense competition surrounding the commercialisation and marketing of nostrums and potions in the Dublin press. Competition was most acute in the cities and towns where a medical marketplace was economically sustainable and there was a clientele willing to buy potions and drugs. The listings in the trade directories for the cities of Dublin and Cork indicate a steady increase in the number of self-styled druggists and apothecaries from the 1780s.[22] As in England, the rise of the druggists was also identified as a problem in the areas better served by regular practitioners. This hostility towards practices dismissed as 'quack' by Dublin medical circles continued into the nineteenth century. Newspapers and 'men considered to hold some rank in the profession'[23] who allowed their names to be used to lend credence to 'quack' claims were targeted. This was not solely a feature of the reform campaign, but continued into the late nineteenth century. In June 1872, in an article entitled 'The Pests of Society', *The Irish Builder* denounced the *Freeman's Journal*, the *Irish Times* and the *Irish Sportsman and Farmer* for continuing to 'publish a filthy class of quack medical advertisements'.[24] Typically, 'quacks' were classed along with moneylenders and gamblers as 'rogues' and 'swindling scoundrels' inflicted upon the public.[25] In the nineteenth century the nomenclature was not confined to the vendor of nostrums but extended to the 'dealer in Mesmerism', homoeopathy, magnetic miracles and the water cure.[26] In their dismissal of these practices and practitioners, authors often identified the inherent 'foreignness' of these treatments. As Jones has shown, exiled French dentists entering the English market struggled with similar xenophobia at the beginning of the nineteenth century (Jones 2007: 85-6). But this hostility was not confined to large urban areas. Dispensary doctors and associated nurses working on the west coast of Ireland were critical of 'unlicenced' practitioners, particularly druggists and bone-setters.[27]

However, while there is evidence of the 'hardening of boundaries' (Brown 2007: 239), as James Bradley has argued in his study of hydropathy, reactions to heterodox medical practices in the nineteenth century were often diverse (Bradley 2002). The publications of Thomas More Madden emphasise the 'fragmented' response of the medical profession and of the nature of medical knowledge when presented with certain heterodox practices (ibid.) More Madden was a member of a medical and literary family; his father was Richard Robert Madden, author of *The United Irishmen, their Lives and Times* (1843–6) and a Fellow of the Royal College of Surgeons of London (Lyons 1978: 74). Having ceased to practice he had a career in the colonial service and eventually was appointed secretary to the Loan Fund Board in Dublin (O'Hart 1915: 302). Thomas was born while his father was in Havana, Cuba. He became a Fellow of the Royal College of Surgeons of London in 1862 and was a highly respected member of the Irish and British medical profession. He specialised in obstetrics and acted as physician to the Mater Misericordiae Hospital, Dublin until his death in 1902 (see Marland 2004). More Madden published widely, and in addition to medical texts he published a genealogy of the O'Madden family (More Madden 1894). He was not particularly hostile to heterodox medicine, and in line with some of his English contemporaries he was willing to endorse hydropathy and published two treatises on European spas (More Madden 1867, 1876). Closer to home, he published his treatise on the *Lucan Spa and Hydropathic as a Modern Health Resort* in Dublin in 1891. Sir Charles Cameron and Sir Dominic Corrigan, among others, are cited as 'highly commending the Lucan Sulphur Spring water' (More Madden 1891: 30–31). Despite the self-confident assertions found in the Irish medical press, by the end of the century medical practitioners remained unsure of the boundaries between orthodoxy and heterodoxy. This is particularly evident in some of More Madden's other publications. In a paper entitled the 'Revival of Old Fallacies bearing on Medicine', read before the Royal Academy of Medicine in Ireland in May 1890 and published in the *Dublin Journal of Medical Science* later that year, More Madden outlined his understanding of the origins of hypnotism, massage and faith healing. His contention was that these 'therapeutic models' 'have been founded on a substructure of truth that outlived the often unconscious exaggerations and delusions with which they were thus intermixed' (More Madden 1890: 22). In this article he characterised each as 'fads' and where possible stressed the foreign elements in their development; hypnotism and the associated magnetism are both portrayed as continental. He was, however, less critical of massage, claiming it was 'useful in certain cases' (ibid.) The success of massage was associated with the activities of Valentine Greatrakes, whose Irish genealogy was conceded although the popularisation of his claims was accredited to a Warwickshire medical practitioner. In the characterisations of these alternative practices, the typical criticisms of faddism, delusions and superstition are present. However, in a series of articles published in the *The Medical Magazine* in London in 1899, More Madden is less certain; instead he claims that the 'alleged marvels of modern hypnotism' and the 'employment of anaesthetics in surgical operations' were known to ancient Irish medical practitioners (More Madden 1899). More Madden was clearly influenced by the escalation of antiquarian interest in ancient Irish texts: he had published a treatise *On the Medical Knowledge of the Ancient Irish* in 1881 and had studied the medical manuscripts housed in Trinity College Dublin and the Royal Irish Academy. Perhaps conscious of his English audience, his intention in *The Medical Magazine* articles was to outline the sophistication and skill of ancient Irish hereditary practitioners and to identify the Irish roots of contemporary medical innovations. His final article in the series identified the efficacy of some of the fourteenth-century Irish *materia medica* and their use in nineteenth-century medicine. More Madden was then engaged with the emerging interest in genealogy and antiquarianism which contributed to the construction of Irish nationhood in the late nineteenth century. Heterodoxy afforded him an opportunity to blend these interests with his studies of therapeutic systems such as hydropathy and hypnotism.

The discussion of elements of folk medicine similarly demonstrated the 'blurred' boundaries between orthodoxy and heterodoxy and medical practitioners' engagement with 'romantic ethnology' in the nineteenth century (Ramsey 1997: 24). Interest in folk medicine was evident among dispensary doctors in addition to contributors to the Irish medical press. The dispensary doctors' interactions with folk practitioners were not uniformly hostile. The local folk practitioner – the bone-setter or wise woman – was not perceived as competition by the salaried dispensary doctor. While bonesetters were characterised as 'avowed opponent[s] of legitimate surgery' (Malone 1879: 385), their presence in a local community did not directly interfere with the income of the doctor. Consequently, dispensary doctors tended to situate the activities of folk practitioners within the local history and ethnography of an area rather than legitimatising them as true competition. Malone's recollections of Biddy Early are illustrative of this point. Malone had never actually met Early and admitted that the source of his information was the local priest. He was persuaded, however, that there was some truth in assertions about her healing powers and even maintained that her remedies corresponded to 'what physicians call an expectant line of treatment' (Malone 1878: 77). The descriptions of Early herself are less flattering. Although Early's cures were appropriated to some extent, her character was denigrated. Two common tropes found in characterisations of Irish 'peasant' society are present; alcoholism and artfulness. Malone draws attention to Early's preference for payment in the form of whiskey rather than money (her rejection of money could be interpreted as a rejection of modernity). The whiskey is then deployed as a means of plying information from the naive public which in turn allows her to display her divining skills. The cunning of the Irish peasant is intertwined with the duplicitous nature of the 'quack' and the 'charlatan'. Despite these character flaws, Early was attended at her death by the local parish priest who witnessed her repentance 'for the life she had led and the scandal she had given' (ibid.) Thus while the cures are legitimatised to some extent, the practitioner is denigrated. It is unclear whether this represents the predictable hostility towards 'untrained' practitioners found elsewhere or a distrust of the Irish peasant. As yet, none of the memoirs of the dispensary doctors analysed identify the absence of a medical education as a danger. Instead, the essential untrustworthiness and fecklessness of the Irish peasant are evoked. The 'idealised' Irish peasant, identified in the writings of participants of the 'cultural revival' such as J.M. Synge is not evident in these treatments (Lane 2004).

There were more explicit attempts to turn 'folk medicine into science' (Timmerman 2001). With some notable exceptions, historians' interrogation of the increased interest in antiquarianism and Irish folk practices in the later nineteenth century have emphasised the rejection of science and the elevation of spiritualism by the architects of the 'Irish Cultural Revival' (Wilson 1991: 95). Certainly the explicit association of the main academic institutions of scientific enquiry with the British interest in Ireland could be a stumbling block. However, while the institutions of science may have represented a problem, the practice of science could lend legitimacy. Echoing More Madden's publications and the responses to hydropathy, numerous descriptions of 'old native remedies' appeared in the *Dublin Journal of Medical Science* in the nineteenth century. In compiling these accounts, some contributors were concerned with preserving and recording ancient practices; Sir William Wilde's accounts of the cures and superstitions of Irish peasants are typical.[28] However, other contributors accompanied descriptions of herbal cures with chemical analysis of their components, thereby attesting to their curative properties. Henry Samuel Purdon's work is representative of this type of treatment. Purdon (1843–1906) was a 'pioneer of dermatology' and was instrumental in the establishment of the Belfast Hospital for Diseases of the Skin (Hall 1970). His interest in 'folk' herbal cures stemmed in part from his dermatological work. He published an article on 'Old Irish Herbal Skin Remedies' in addition to a general piece entitled 'Notes on Old Native Remedies' (Purdon 1895, 1898). In these articles he attested to the continued popularity of an individual herbal cure which was accompanied by a 'scientific' commentary. His treatment of burdock root was typical:

> Everyone living in the country, at least in the north-east of Ireland, is familiar with the appearance of burdock still largely used ... as a decoction to 'purify the blood'. Formerly a tincture of the seeds of burdock made with wine was taken for sciatica. Burdock is a diuretic and sudorific. Messrs Trimble and MacFarland (*American Journal of Pharmacy* 1888) have found in the seeds a bitter principle which is a glucoside; the root is also rich in potassium salts, which may account for its curative action in psoriasis, gout and rheumatism. (Purdon 1895: 214)

This positivism and scientism can also be seen in the tendency to endorse the pharmacopoeia of Irish folk practitioners found in the articles of the *Journal of the Royal Society of Antiquaries of Ireland*. These assessments of herbal 'cures' differed from the antiquarian accounts of traditional cures, which were mainly descriptive accounts of practices and were in some instances accompanied by patients' testimonies of their success.[29]

Conclusion

The writings on medical practices delineated as 'folk', 'native', 'quack' and 'charlatan' found in Irish medical and literary journals in the nineteenth century emphasise the constructed nature of the boundaries between orthodox and heterodox medical knowledge and practice, and the absence of uniformity of medical knowledge. The boundaries between orthodox and heterodox medical practices remained blurred in the nineteenth century and this was not unique to Ireland. Nor was there a uniform reaction to heterodox practises. Some practitioners, who self-consciously situated themselves within 'the faculty',[30] displayed hostility towards the archetypal nostrum vendor and 'charlatan', and advocates of the water cure, hypnotism and magnetism. However, as the case of hydropathy clearly indicates, biomedical practitioners were invoked to lend sanction and legitimacy. As other essays in this volume show, there are instances of collusion with biomedical models.

Similarly, reactions to 'folk healing' varied; the construction of 'folk' medical practices and practitioners received a different treatment. In the writings of the dispensary doctors, who operated in districts poorly served by 'regular' practitioners and whose income was largely derived from state salaries rather than private practice, literary treatments of 'folk' practices could be less polemic in tone (Ramsey 1997: 27). The folk doctor was not always perceived to be a significant commercial threat. Indeed the folk healer was in greater opposition with the local priest who engaged in his own process of rationalisation which had started before the Great Famine (Ó Héalaí 1991). The practices of folk healers were more closely associated with the revival and rediscovery of Irish traditions. Among elite men, such as More Madden and Purdon, interest in the efficacy of traditional herbal cures overlapped with antiquarianism and attempts to revive Irish language, dance and literature. The extent to which these attitudes were shared by patients is as yet unclear. Among patients, herbal cures remained popular and effective. The apparent confirmation of their efficacy through scientific analysis legitimised their use through the adoption of methodological approaches associated with 'professionalisation'. This allowed orthodox practitioners to prescribe treatments that occupied a secure place within a community's medical repertoire (Gijswijt-Hofstra, Marland and de Waardt 1997: 7–8) and also provided the practice of science with a place within the cultural movements of the late nineteenth century.

Notes

1. For a detailed study of the events, see Bourke (1999).
2. For a discussion of patients' attitudes, see Porter (1992) and Ernst (2002).
3. For a useful overview of the historiography, see Malcolm and Jones (1999).
4. See the following articles: 'Medical Reform' (17 March 1858); 'Medical Legislation' (31 March 1858); 'The Reform Mania' (14 April 1858); 'The Medical Act' (28 July 1858), all in *Dublin Medical Press*.
5. Source: 'Return of the Name of Each Person in Each Year since 24th of June 1791, Who Has Been Examined by the Governor and Director of the Apothecaries' Hall in Dublin, and Who Has Received a Certificate of his Qualification to Become an Apprentice, an Assistant Journeyman and to Open a Shop and Practise as an Apothecary in Ireland', British Parliamentary Papers 1829 (235) 22.
6. Ibid.

7. For an account of the difficulties the apothecaries encountered, see Fleetwood (1983: 90–91).
8. 'Pharmacy in Ireland', *Dublin Medical Press*, 25 August 1858.
9. For an assessment of the development of Victorian Dublin, see Daly (1984), Prunty (2000) and Brady and Simms (2001).
10. For an account of other famines, see Crawford (1989).
11. Margaret Pelling and Charles Webster (1979) developed this definition to 'take into account all practitioners involved in dispensing medical care'. They argue that the focus on 'university-educated practitioners' or on those 'involved with the organized bodies of surgeons and apothecaries' excludes the class of practitioners who may have been dominant in certain regions.
12. Carlow town had one practitioner per 1,668 patients, while Kilkenny city had one per 827 patients.
13. In 1891 the doctor/patient ratio in each county was: Cork, 1 to 2,227; Kerry, 1 to 3,380; Carlow, 1 to 3,824; and Kilkenny, 1 to 3,629.
14. Table 3.1: Doctor/Patient Ratio, Ireland, 1841 and 1851.

	1841	1851
Cork County	3,876	6,227
Donegal County	5,024	8,798
Kerry County	3,867	9,927
Mayo	9,259	13,071

15. 'Oppression of the Dispensary Surgeon', *Dublin Medical Press*, 1 May 1839.
16. Delgany Dispensary Minute Book, 19 February 1852. MS 16411, Hodson Papers, National Library of Ireland.
17. 'Oppression of Dispensary System', *Dublin Medical Press*, 1 May 1839.
18. For example, see Delgany Dispensary Minute Book, 12 March 1854. MS 16411, Hodson Papers, National Library of Ireland.
19. 'Cork Dispensary: Salaries of Medical Officers' (12 May 1858); 'Cork Union: Salaries of Dispensary Officers' (7 July 1858), both in *Dublin Medical Press*.
20. 'Is Cod-Liver Oil a Medicine?' *Dublin Medical Press*, September 1858.
21. The term 'folklore' was defined by the British antiquarian William John Thoms; see Ramsey (1997: 25).
22. Sources: Anon. (1786) and Lucas (1967).
23. 'Liaisons Dangereuse – Quacks and their Patrons', *Dublin Medical Press*, 3 April 1839.
24. 'The Pests of Society', *The Irish Builder*, 1 June 1872.
25. Ibid.
26. 'The Water-cure – Mr Claridge', *Dublin University Magazine*, June 1842.
27. For examples, see 'Memorandum on Unqualified Medical Practice in Ireland' in *Report as to the Practice of Medicine and Surgery by Unqualified*

persons in the United Kingdom, British Parliamentary Papers 1910 [Cd. 5422] 43: 65–85.

28. See Wilde's series of articles, 'Irish Popular Superstitions', published between May 1849 and May 1850 in *Dublin University Magazine*.
29. See, e.g., Letter from J. Dillon to J. Todd, 1 February 1848. Papers of Eugene O'Curry (1796–1862), University College Dublin Archives.
30. Ibid.

References

Anon. 1786. *The Gentleman's and Citizen's Almanack*. Dublin: Stewart & Hopes.

Athill, L. 2007. *Recollections of an Irish Doctor*. Whitegate: Ballinakella Press.

Barrington, R. 2000. *Health, Medicine and Politics in Ireland 1900–1970*. Dublin: Institute of Public Administration.

Bivins, R. 2007. *Alternative Medicine. A History*. Oxford: Oxford University Press.

Bourke, A. 1995. 'Reading a Women's Death: Colonial Text and Oral Tradition in Nineteenth-century Ireland', *Feminist Studies* 21: 553–85.

Bourke, A. 1999. *The Burning of Bridget Cleary*. London: Pimlico.

Brady, J. and A. Simms (eds). 2001. *Dublin Through Space and Time (c.900–1900)*. Dublin: Four Courts Press.

Bradley, J. 2002. 'Medicine on the Margins? Hydropathy and Orthodoxy in Britain, 1840–1860', in W. Ernst (ed.) *Plural Medicine, Tradition and Modernity, 1800–2000*. London and New York: Routledge.

Brown, M. 2007. 'Medicine, Quackery and the Free Market: The War against Morrison's Pills and the Construction of the Medical Profession, c.1830–c.1850', in M. Jenner and P. Wallis (eds), *Medicine and the Market in England and its Colonies, c.1450–c.1850*. Basingstoke: Palgrave Macmillan.

Brunton, D. 1999. The Problems of Implementation: the Failure and Success of Public Vaccination against Smallpox in Ireland, 1840–1873', in E. Malcom and G. Jones (eds), *Medicine, Disease and the State in Ireland, 1650–1940*. Cork: Cork University Press.

Clyde, T. 2003. *Irish Literary Magazines*. Dublin: Irish Academic Press.

Cooter, R. (ed.) 1988. *Studies in the History of Alternative Medicine*. Basingstoke: Macmillan in association with St. Anthony's College, Oxford.

Crawford, M. (ed.) 1989. *Famine: The Irish Experience, 900–1900*. Edinburgh: John Donald.

Daly, M.E. 1984. *Dublin, the Deposed Capital: A Social and Economic History, 1860–1914*. Cork: Cork University Press.

______. 2006. *The Slow Failure: Population Decline and Independent Ireland, 1920–1973*. Madison, Wisconsin: University of Wisconsin Press.

Digby, A. 1999. *The Evolution of British General Practice 1850–1948*. Oxford: Clarendon Press.

______. 2002. *Making a Medical Living: Doctors and Patients in the English Market for Medicine, 1720–1911*. Cambridge: Cambridge University Press.

Ernst, W. 2002. 'Plural Medicine, Tradition and Modernity: Historical and Contemporary Perspectives: Views from Below and from Above', in W. Ernst (ed.) *Plural Medicine, Tradition and Modernity, 1800–2000*. London and New York: Routledge.

Fleetwood, J. 1983. *The History of Medicine*. Dublin: Skellig Press.

Froggatt, P. 1989. 'The Response of the Medical Profession to the Great Famine', in M.E. Crawford (ed.) *Famine: The Irish Experience, 900–1900*. Edinburgh: John Donald.

Geary, L.M. 2004. *Medicine and Charity in Ireland, 1718–1851*. Dublin: University College Dublin Press.

Guinnane, T. 1997. *The Vanishing Ireland: Households, Migration and the Rural Economy in Ireland, 1850–1914*. Princeton: Princeton University Press.

Hall, R. 1970. 'History of Dermatology in Northern Ireland', *British Journal of Dermatology* 83: 690–97.

Hoff, J. and M. Yeates. 2000. *The Cooper's Wife is Missing: The Trials of Bridget Cleary*. New York: Basic Books.

Gijswijt-Hofstra, M., H. Marland and H. de Waardt (eds). 1997. *Illness and Healing Alternatives in Western Europe*. London and New York: Routledge.

Jones, C. 2007. 'French Dentists and English Teeth in the Long Eighteenth Century: A Tale of Two Cities and One Dentist', in R. Bivins and J.V. Pickstone (eds), *Medicine, Madness and Social History*. Basingstoke: Palgrave Macmillan.

Jones, G. 2006. 'Medicine and the Making of the Irish Middle Class: Medicine and Migration, 1860–1911', unpublished paper delivered at the Economic and Social History Society of Ireland Annual Conference, Belfast, 17–18 November 2006.

Kelly, J. 2005. 'Health for Sale: Doctors, Mountebanks and Quacks and the Purveying if Medication in Eighteenth-Century Ireland', unpublished paper presented at the workshop 'Practices and Culture of Care in Irish Medical History', University of Warwick, 2 June 2005.

Kirkpatrick, T.C. 1915. 'An Account of the Irish Medical Periodicals', *Dublin Journal of Medical Science* (140) 1–13.

Lane, L. 2004. "There are Compensations in the Congested Districts for their Poverty": AE and the Idealized Peasant of the Agricultural Co-operative

Movement', in B.T. Fitzsimon and J.H. Murphy (eds), *The Irish Revival Reappraised*. Dublin: Four Courts Press.

Loudon, I. 1987. 'The Vile Race of Quacks with which this Country is Infested' in W.F. Bynum and R. Porter (eds), *Medical Fringe and Medical Orthodoxy, 1750–1850*. London: Croom Helm.

______. 1996. *Medical Care and the General Practitioner, 1750–1850*. Oxford: Clarendon Press.

Lucas, R. 1967. 'The Cork Directory for the Year 1787', *Journal of the Cork Historical and Archaeological Society* 72(216): 135–57.

Lyons, J.B. 1978. *Brief Lives of Irish Doctors*. Dublin: Blackwater Press.

MacDonagh, O. 1989. 'Ideas and Institutions' in W.E. Vaughan (ed.) *A New History of Ireland: Ireland under the Union, vol.* 5. Oxford: Clarendon Press.

McKay, A. 2005. 'Medicine and Ethics in the Indo-Tibetan Himalayas', unpublished paper delivered at University of Warwick, 26 October 2005.

Malcolm, E. and G. Jones. 1999. 'Introduction: An Anatomy of Irish Medical History', in E. Malcolm and G. Jones (eds), *Medicine, Disease and the State in Ireland*. Cork: Cork University Press.

Malone, M.J. 1878. 'Recollections of a Country Dispensary', *Irish Monthly* 6: 72–79

______. 1879. 'Doctoring Under Difficulties', *Irish Monthly* 7: 383–88.

Marland, H. 2004. 'Madden, Thomas More (1844–1902)', *Oxford Dictionary of National Biography*. Oxford: Oxford University Press.

More Madden, T. 1867. *The Spas of Belgium, Germany, Switzerland France and Italy*. Dublin: M.H. Gill & Son.

______. 1876. *The Principal Health Resorts of Europe and Africa for the Treatment of Chronic Diseases*. London: Churchill.

______. 1890. 'Revival of Old Fallacies Bearing on Medicine', *Dublin Journal of Medical Science* 90: 22–41.

______. 1891. *Lucan Spa and Hydropathic as a Modern Health Resort*. Dublin: M.H. Gill & Son.

______. 1894. *Genealogical, Historical and Family Records of the O'Maddens of Hy-Many*. Dublin: W. Powell.

______. 1899. 'Ancient Irish Medicine: Its Culture and Practice', *The Medical Magazine* 8: 610–16, 676–82, 896–905, 990–96.

Mortimer, I. 2007. 'The Rural Medical Marketplace in Southern England c.1570–1720', in M. Jenner and P. Wallis (eds), *Medicine and the Market in England and Its Colonies, c.1450–c.1850*. Basingstoke: Palgrave Macmillan.

Ó Gráda, C. 1994. *Ireland: A New Economic History, 1780–1939*. Oxford: Oxford University Press.

O'Hart, J. 1915. *Irish Pedigrees: Or the Origins and Stem of the Irish Nation*, Vol. 2. New York: M'Glashan & Gill.

Ó Héalaí, P. 1991. 'Priest Versus Healer: The Legend of the Priest's Stricken Horse', *Béaloideas* 59: 171–88.

O'Neill, T.P. 1973. 'Fever and Public Health in Pre-famine Ireland', *Journal of the Royal Society of Antiquaries of Ireland* 103: 1–34.

Peeters, E. 2008. 'Inventing Medical Authority: Natural Therapy and Medical Modernisation in Belgium', unpublished paper presented at the workshop 'The Medical Marketplace and Medical Tradition: Interfaces between Orthodox, Alternative and Folk Practice in the Nineteenth and Twentieth Centuries', University College Dublin, 1 February 2008.

Pelling, M. and C. Webster. 1979. 'Medical Practitioners', in C. Webster (ed.) *Health, Medicine and Mortality in the Sixteenth Century*. Cambridge: Cambridge University Press.

Porter, R. (ed.), 1992. *The Popularization of Medicine, 1650–1850*. London and New York: Routledge.

______. 2003. *Quacks: Fakers and Charlatans in English Medicine*. Stroud: Tempus.

Prior, P. 2006. 'Roasting a Man Alive: The Case of Mary Reilly, Criminal Lunatic', *Éire-Ireland* 41: 169–91.

Prunty, J. 2000. *Dublin Slums 1800–1925: A Study in Urban Geography*. Dublin: Irish Academic Press.

Purdon, H. 1895. 'Notes on Old Native Remedies', *Dublin Journal of Medical Science* 100: 214–18

______. 1898. 'Old Irish "Herbal" Skin Remedies', *Dublin Journal of Medical Science* 106: 27–31.

Ramsey, M. 1997. 'Magical Healing, Witchcraft and Elite Discourse in Eighteenth- and Nineteenth-century France', in M. Gijswijt-Hofstra, H. Marland and H. de Waardt (eds), *Illness and Healing Alternatives*. London and New York: Routledge.

Timmerman, C. 2001. 'Rationalizing "Folk Medicine" in Interwar Germany: Faith, Business and Science at "Dr. Mathaus & Co"', *Social History of Medicine* 14: 459–82.

Vaughan, W.E. 1989. 'Ireland c.1870', in W.E. Vaughan (ed.) *A New History of Ireland: Ireland under the Union, vol.* 5. Oxford: Clarendon Press.

Vaughan, W.E. and A.J. Fitzpatrick. 1978. *Irish Historical Statistics: Population, 1821*–1971. Dublin: Royal Irish Academy.

Wilson, J.W. 1991. 'Natural Science and Irish Culture', *Éire-Ireland* 26: 92–103.

Chapter 4

Folk Healing in Rural Wales: The Use of Wool Measuring

Susan Philpin

Introduction

Wool measuring refers to a particular type of folk healing described in Welsh folk literature from the late nineteenth and early twentieth centuries but rooted in antiquity, which has survived in parts of rural mid Wales to the present day. Although the folk literature from earlier periods describes the practice in relation to a number of illnesses, the most common form of illness for which wool measuring is currently sought is the condition that people in the communities studied define as 'depression'[1] or, to use the Welsh expression, *clefyd-y-galon,* being 'sick at heart'. This chapter explores the ways in which the culture of a particular community may influence people's understanding of the nature of illness and thus their healing choices. Following an account of the methods used in my study of this practice, I will outline the wool measuring procedure as it is currently practised in the communities studied. I will then briefly describe the communities where wool measuring persists. Finally, the various elements comprising the process of wool measuring will be explored in terms of their meaning(s) to the people involved: healers and sufferers.[2]

Background

There is much in the folk-healing literature from various parts of the world involving the use of ritual measurement in healing. For example, Hancock (1873), Owen (1887), Williams (1888), Davies (1911), Peate (1924), Winstanley and Rose (1926), Jones (1930) and Evans (1937) all describe the practice in several parts of late nineteenth- and early twentieth-century Wales, with Davies, writing just before the Second World War, noting that the practice is 'very prevalent in Wales even today' (Davies 1938: 166). Elsewhere, Westropp (1911) refers to the practice of 'head-measuring' to 'close the skull' and cure headaches in County Clare, Ireland, earlier this century, and St Clair (1971) reports the contemporary use of the 'ribbon of comfort' in Ulster to measure and enclose the pain of a headache. Nordland (1961), meanwhile, alludes to wool measuring for diagnostic purposes by a 'wise woman' in Oslo earlier this century, though it is not clear what form this measuring takes or if it is also used for healing.

Ritual measurement is rooted in antiquity, although it is clear that such practices have undergone changes over time. Thomas (1971) refers to girdle measuring in the fifteenth and sixteenth centuries in England and throughout Europe, and Thorndike (1923) also describes the practice in medieval Europe. Hand notes that 'the measuring of people to learn, first of all, whether they are afflicted, and, secondly, to divest them of disease if they have one, apparently is a practice going back to the time of Pliny the Elder, if not before' (Hand 1980: 107).

Descriptive accounts of wool measuring in the Welsh folk literature are essentially very similar although there are some notable variations. Jones (1930), for example, refers to a number of reports of the practice in various parts of mid Wales and describes the method used by a Wesleyan preacher who was said to have cured 'hundreds of persons', as follows:

> his process was to place one end of the yarn on the elbow of the patient, measuring to the tip of the middle finger. Then the patient, or his representative (it seems it was not necessary for the sufferer to attend), took hold of the piece of the yarn and pulled. If the yarn lengthened, the patient was understood to be suffering from the complaint; if it contracted (in a second measuring probably), then the patient was said to be suffering from some other disease. If the yarn showed the presence of the heart complaint, (i.e. *heart sickness* in the figurative sense), it was tied around the patient's arm until a cure was accomplished. (ibid.: 131).

In addition to the measuring ritual, Jones describes the following potion that the patient would in some cases be given to drink: 'A piece of hot steel, weighing half a pound, is heated red hot and placed in half a cupful of beer and left in it. A sixpenny worth of saffron is infused in a cupful of boiling water, which is then mixed with the beer' (ibid.)

Although Jones's description of the measurement process was the most common method, the literature also refers to various practices regarding what was done with the wool after measuring. Tying the wool around a part of the body is mentioned in some of the descriptions, and different parts of the body were used. For example, Hancock notes that, 'After the existence and nature of the complaint was thus determined, the thread was made into a skein and put around the neck of the patient' (Hancock 1873: 329). Similarly, Winstanley and Rose (1926) tell of a *dynes hysbys*[3] in Aberystwyth using grey wool tied around the wrist as a charm to ward off ill luck.

Folk healers described in the Welsh literature usually had other jobs in addition to their healing role and their healing ability tended to run in families. It was also very common for them to treat animals as well as humans, and they were often called upon for other problems besides illness, such as finding lost or stolen property, discovering why butter would not churn, divination and counteracting the supposed effects of witchcraft against both people and animals.

Conditions Treated by Wool Measuring

The nineteenth-century Welsh folk literature describes a number of different conditions treated by wool measuring, the most common of which is *clefyd-y-galon*, literally 'sickness or disease of the heart'. However, the term appears to be used in a variety of ways: Jones notes that 'it does not appear that the complaint is what is commonly known as heart disease' (Jones 1930:130), while Owen (1887) notes that *clefyd-y-galon* may be translated as 'heart disease' or as 'love sickness' and cites an example of wool measuring being used to cure the latter condition with success.

Jones (1930) also observes that wool measuring was used to treat *clwy'r edau wlan*, 'disease of the woollen thread', thus naming the condition in terms of its required treatment. It appears that sometimes *clefyd-y-galon* and *clwy'r edau wlan* are used interchangeably to describe the same condition. Williams, however, describes *clwy'r edau wlan* as 'jaundice and other complaints of the liver and spleen' (Williams 1888: 327). Similarly, Hancock describes *clwy'r edef wlan*[4] thus: 'The symptoms resembled jaundice. Also where persons had been for some time suffering from great debility and prostration of the nervous system and unable to account for their illness, resort was laid to the *edef wlan*' (Hancock 1873: 328). More recently, in his study of the people of the Dyfi Basin in northern Powys, Peate refers to a 'charmer' who treated 'scores of people for jaundice which is known in all its forms as *clwy'r edau wlan*, the woollen yarn disease, since the remedy was to measure a piece of yarn from the elbow to the tip of the middle finger of the patient' (Peate 1924: 178).

Wool measuring was also seen as appropriate for 'wasting diseases' and consumption. For example, Jones refers to a disease in Montgomeryshire that was cured by wool measuring and described as 'a kind of *diciau* (Eng. decay, consumption), and was believed to be due to witchcraft' (Jones 1930: 131). Similarly, Owen (1887) describes woollen thread sickness as referring to consumption. And Evans, in her account of 'magicians' in Cardiganshire using wool measuring, notes that the process was supposed to be a certain cure for 'people suffering from Heart Diseases or Consumption' (Evans 1937: 57).

The folk literature suggests that the practice of wool measuring was more widely distributed and known about in the past and that folk healers included wool measuring in their repertoire of healing methods rather than there being particular healers who used wool measuring exclusively. This contrasts with the present situation where wool measuring is the sole healing method of the healers in the study. Particular aspects of the wool measuring process – such as familial links between healers, the cubit as a unit of measurement, and the prescription of potions – have persisted to the present day and will be discussed later. However, while in the past the terms *clefyd-y-galon* and *clwy'r-edef-wlan* referred to a wide range of what were described as mainly physical conditions – heart disease, consumption, jaundice, nervous debility – today these terms are used to describe 'depression'.

Methods

Data for this ethnographic study of wool measuring were generated from direct participant and non-participant observation of the process of wool measuring (on one occasion I had my wool measured), with additional data being drawn from both conversations and unstructured interviews with those involved. The study also included the analysis of different types of documentary material. First (with permission and attention to the maintenance of anonymity), letters written to the healers in the study requesting healing or expressing gratitude for healing were examined. In addition, nineteenth-century Welsh folk literature pertaining to popular belief concerning healing, provided not only a background to the study but also a rich source of data and allowed temporal comparisons of healing practices. Both types of document were intriguing in terms of their content and also in terms of what they represented and how they were used (Scott 1990; Prior 2003).

The study also drew on the knowledge and practice of key informants. I use the term informants to indicate that my study was informed by particular people within this cultural group (Spradley 1980). The key informants were people who practised and received wool measuring; in addition, they were people who had witnessed wool measuring and/or lived in a locality where wool measuring is practised. The number of healers interviewed and observed was small; although six people practising wool measuring in rural Wales at the time of the study were identified, of these six, only four agreed to take part in the study. Three of the healers interviewed were female and one was male, their ages ranging from forty-eight to eighty-two years. All were natives of rural mid Wales and all spoke Welsh as their first language.

Twelve sufferers and five witnesses who were community members were also interviewed. Of the twelve sufferers interviewed, three of the subjects were under the age of thirty; the other nine were over fifty-five. There were seven females to five males and all subjects except one either lived in the same village as the healer or within a five-mile radius. The sufferers were all Welsh-speaking and predominantly from skilled manual occupations. Individuals who had witnessed healing and/or lived in communities where this practice took place were additional sources of information about the ways in which the practice was perceived by the community.

The study was underpinned by reflexivity involving awareness that, in addition to influencing the behaviour and relationships within the group being studied, my 'self' as a researcher was also being changed by these relationships; and that moreover both these influences and changes constitute the data (Davies 1999). Reflexivity also demands that aspects of my personal biography which influence my identity and position as a stranger or an insider within the group need to be recognised and brought to the fore.

First, my ethnic identity. On one level, as English-Australian by birth and upbringing, this marginalised me in a rural Welsh community. However, ethnic identity is not always straightforward and in my case it is also influenced by historical family connections with rural mid Wales (although not with the communities studied), which inculcated strong emotional links and indeed feelings of belonging to this part of the world and its people. Ethnicity of course also involves language, and I was aware that my status as a non-Welsh speaker was also marginalising. A further influential aspect of my biography is that, as a qualified nurse, I am sensitive to the fact that my earlier enculturation into biomedical education influences my understanding of the condition described as 'depression'. In biomedical terms this refers to a particular, although often diffuse, collection of symptoms, treated by medical (including psychotherapeutic) interventions. Attempts to discover what this condition meant to the sufferers required a conscious bracketing of the biomedical meaning of the term. In addition, my enculturation into biomedical science also engendered considerable scepticism in me towards wool measuring as a therapeutic intervention, which also necessitated conscious bracketing throughout the study.

The Wool Measuring Procedure

Wool measurement, sometimes referred to as 'healing with the woollen yarn', is a method of healing that, unusually, does not involve the application of any direct treatment to the sufferer. Rather, it consists of a particular form of self-measurement, undertaken by the healer on the sufferer's behalf. Although there are variations, the following method used by one of the female healers in my study demonstrates the main elements described in the folk literature[5] and by witnesses' accounts of older (now deceased) healers.

An essential preliminary requirement to wool measurement is precise information regarding the sufferer's full name and date of birth. Once these details are noted, the healer then takes hold of one end of a pre-determined length of wool, the other end of which is firmly attached to a solid object. They then proceed to 'measure' the length of this thread of wool three times against the distance from their inner elbow to the tip of their middle finger, a distance that they define as a 'cubit'. Sound health is indicated if the length of wool corresponds, in each person's measuring process, to three cubits; if, however, all is not well with an individual, the healer finds the thread to be either shorter or longer in length than three cubits. The severity of the illness is indicated by the amount of discrepancy between the actual and desired length of the wool. The same thread of wool is used for each measuring performed on each of the healer's clients until the yarn becomes too worn to use. After an apparently arbitrary period, the healer repeats the measuring process, sometimes three or four times a day, the length of the wool informing them of the sufferer's progress. The measuring continues, for each individual, until the thread reaches the correct length, indicating that the sufferer is cured. Thus, it appears that this measuring procedure encompasses both 'diagnosis' and 'treatment' of the sufferer's problem.

Sufferers do not necessarily have to be in the presence of the healer physically while their wool is being measured, or even to be aware that measurement is taking place. It is enough for a request for healing to be made (either by the sufferer or on their behalf by a relative or friend) by telephone or letter. Sufferers also included animals: one healer said that she had healed a pony and a dog that were 'pining' by wool measurement. Similar animal healing events were also recounted by other witnesses and are also described in the folk literature. None of the healers interviewed charged for their services, although one of them made the acceptability of a 'donation' clear to prospective clients.

Communities Where Wool Measuring Persists

In order to understand the meaning of this healing practice, it is necessary to situate it in the social and historical context of the type of community where it still persists. The healers in my study practised in villages characterised by geographical isolation due to the mountainous terrain. Older informants noted that in earlier years their isolation had made access to medical help difficult, hence the need for locally based folk healers. For example, a 79-year-old woman described a local folk healer from her youth (in this case one who was able to stop bleeding in addition to wool measuring) who was often called out for farming accidents because 'they needed someone on the spot, there was no time to get a doctor'.

In addition to their geographic isolation, these villages were less affected than many others in rural Wales by outward and inward migration,[6] which may have contributed to the maintenance of traditional beliefs (albeit with some modifications) and practices in this community. The communities were close-knit, their members bound by multiple ties of kinship, affinity, neighbourliness, chapel membership and, significantly, the Welsh language. All but one of my informants were native Welsh speakers, with Welsh being the first language they had learned, the language through which (in most cases) they had received their primary education, and the language they used in everyday conversation. There is a complex interrelationship between language, nationality and culture in Wales (see Jones 1993; Bowie 1993) and it would appear that the Welsh language was a key factor in framing villagers' perceived national-cum-ethnic identity, both in terms of reinforcing 'belonging' and defining cultural boundaries. Moreover, Welsh was found to play a very important role in the transmission of cultural knowledge and traditions, including knowledge about wool measuring.

However, despite the fact that cultural knowledge was transmitted through these strong social networks, informants (apart from the healers themselves) were hard pressed to explain how they came to know about wool measuring. That is, they were unable to be specific about either the source of the knowledge or the channel through which it was communicated, frequently commenting that 'wool measuring was always around us, we grew up knowing it was there for us'. They generally felt that wool measuring was 'common knowledge', something that everyone in the village knew about. Informants commented that wool measuring would be talked about in the context of enquiring about people's health wherever meetings took place – in the home, at family gatherings, in the pub, outside the school gate, in the village shops and in the chapel. The overwhelming impression I gained was of the very ordinariness of this folk knowledge. The healers' knowledge of wool measuring and their ability to heal, as with folk healers in the literature, was 'passed on' from parent or grandparent or from an older person in the village to the next generation. These links between generations of healers also re-emphasise the healers' connectedness to their local communities.

Wool Measuring as a Therapeutic Process

The following analysis of the healing process seeks to explore its meaning to those involved. Wool measuring appears to fit Helman's description of symbolic healing, in that it 'does not rely on any physical or pharmacological treatments for its efficacy, but rather on language, ritual and the manipulation of powerful cultural symbols' (Helman 2007: 274). It is useful to explore the symbolism and ritual inherent in wool measuring through its various stages, including variation in the ways in which different practitioners perform the procedure and in healers' and sufferers' perceptions of the efficacy of the practice. As a starting point the nature of the illnesses treated by wool measuring will be explored.

The Nature of the Illnesses Treated by Wool Measuring

The illnesses for which present-day sufferers and their families seek recourse to wool measuring are not easily classified or 'cured' by orthodox medicine. The main category of illness for which wool measuring is currently sought is 'depression', and this was referred to by all my informants: sufferers, healers and witnesses. However, the term 'depression' was used by informants to include a variety of related conditions such as anxiety, 'nerves', 'breakdowns' and being 'run-down'. Depression appeared to be used as a catch-all term used to describe sufferers' experiences of not feeling 'right'. In addition, sufferers often described their illness in terms of how they were physically experiencing this condition, using physical terminology such as 'something pressing on you', 'something is pressing on your heart', and 'when the pain is hanging heavy on you'. Informants' descriptions of their own or other sufferers' behaviour would often include the need to withdraw from social and work commitments, sometimes actually taking to their beds.

The biomedical understanding of depression similarly includes a moulding of emotional distress into mainly physical symptoms, a process known as somatisation (Kleinman 1980; Helman 2007). For instance, Helman notes that depressed patients may complain of 'a variety of diffuse, and often changeable physical symptoms: such as "tired all the time", headaches, palpitations, weight loss, dizziness, vague aches and pains, and so on' (Helman 2007: 260). This list of physical symptoms echoes to some extent the variety of conditions described earlier in the review of the folk literature with which people consulted wool measurers and may shed some light on the diffuse nature of their complaints. The previously noted old Welsh term for depression, *clefyd-y-galon*, is intriguing in its translation as 'heart sickness', or as some informants said 'to be sick at heart', in that it suggests a physical experience of an emotional state (cf. Good 1977). It also implies a perception of the heart and spirit as one, as opposed to Cartesian distinctions between mind and body. Notions of unity of heart and spirit (or mind and body) are also inherent in the idea, gained from this study, that informants were clear that it was the whole person who needed healing, rather than a collection of symptoms. This is exemplified by the explanation from one of the sufferers who had undergone successful wool measuring for depression, anaemia and a 'generally poor condition': 'It didn't matter which she was treating me for, anaemia, depression, whatever, because she was treating *me* the person, not the condition'. This resonates with Kleinman's (1986) suggestion that indigenous healers' skills lie in their ability to treat 'illness' rather than cure disease; they are able to make people feel better.

In similar vein to the folk literature, a number of healers in the study also used the expression *clwyr'r-edau-wlan* ('disease of the woollen yarn') to describe depression. A further indication of the looseness of the folk classification of depressive illness, and indeed the mixing of physical and emotional diagnoses, is the fact that, as in the folk literature, informants often described jaundice as occurring with, or following on from, depression, and this was seen by many as being equally amenable to wool measuring. For instance, a sufferer in his sixties recalled how his grandmother sought wool measuring for him as a child if he 'looked a bit yellow'; he presumed this must have been for some kind of jaundice which, he thought, was more prevalent at that time. It is possible, however, that 'looking yellow' may also be another depiction of depression. The same informant commented that a term for depression in the dialect of North Wales is *y-melyn*, which he glossed as 'they have got the yellow on them' (not a literal translation). Another informant in his early seventies, who had been healed by wool measuring and also often watched it done on others, commented that: 'depression, or *clefyd-y-galon* as we call it, often followed jaundice'. In this case, 'depression' may have been lassitude following a debilitating infection.

Some healers also described being able to treat abdominal pain associated with gallstones and other 'stomach' complaints. The link between gallstones and jaundice may also be relevant. One sufferer, the daughter of a healer, commented that 'I don't go to the doctor any more with stomach pain, I just ask Mam'. Wool measuring was, on three occasions, reported as being used to treat 'failure to thrive'. For instance the sixty-year-old man described earlier had also been measured as a very young baby, at his grandmother's insistence, because of failure to thrive. His grandmother had been adamant that the measuring had saved his life. There are interesting parallels here with Hand's observations concerning the measuring of children elsewhere in Europe where 'measuring was believed to ensure health and well being, particularly if the child were frail or sickly' (Hand 1980: 108). The use of wool measuring for failure to thrive also echoes the wasting diseases and consumption sometimes referred to in the folk literature.

The Setting of Healing

It is problematic to speak of the 'setting' in which healing took place as the sufferer was not necessarily present for the healing, or even aware that they were being measured. However, out of the twelve sufferers interviewed, four of them did visit the healer's home for healing so it does merit examination. Moreover, the measuring takes place in healers' homes regardless of where the sufferer happens to be. The healers that I visited did their measuring in their living rooms in very ordinary, homely surroundings, with the pet dog running around and grandchildren coming in and out, which emphasises the aforementioned ordinariness of the healing and also the shared values and understandings between healer and sufferer.

In one setting I was particularly aware of the anachronism of the scenario where the wool that was manipulated for this very ancient healing method was anchored to an old transistor radio. This healer explained that if it was attached to the radio it reminded her of her 'patients' each time she went past. She said that the woman who had taught her attached her wool to her clock, another healer attached it to the back of an old oak chair, and one informant discussing a deceased healer described how the man had attached the wool to a nail behind the door and strode towards it as it was measured. On reflection, it seems that all of them were using what was appropriate for their particular circumstances. That is, while the old oak chair or clock were part of the cultural accoutrements of earlier healers, the transistor radio as an anchorage point was apposite for today's healer. It is, perhaps, an illustration of the ways in which traditional practices are adapted to or are embedded in everyday life.

The Taking of Sufferers' Details

Precise information regarding each sufferer's full name and date of birth was an essential preliminary requirement to wool measurement in all the cases studied. Some healers required more precise information about dates of birth than others, and some also required the sufferer's exact place of residence. For example, one healer commented that he must know 'their full name and exactly when they were born – right down to the month – and their address, even the county'.

The requirement for this information, particularly people's place of residence, is intriguing and suggestive of the ways in which close-knit, rural communities are structured. That is, they are based on knowledge about people's families and where individuals 'fit' in the community (indeed, informants often asked me where 'my people' came from). Obviously, this suggestion does not apply in the same way to outsiders seeking treatment, but there may still be an attempt by the healer to 'place' these sufferers. In addition, details about sufferers appeared to give the healer something to focus on, all the more necessary in view of the fact that some sufferers were not present to be measured. For instance one of the healers said that once he had the sufferer's details he would 'think about them very hard, forget about everything else'. Similarly, another informant described a deceased healer who, when given the details of absent sufferers by a surrogate, would close his eyes saying 'let me have a look at them'.

What Happens During Measuring?

It is difficult to apprehend from either my study or the folk literature what is actually being measured. Neither sufferer nor healer could explain this and both were apparently unconcerned, which highlights the importance given over to performative elements in forms of ritual measurement. When questioned as to what, specifically, was being measured, most of the sufferers replied that it was 'their wool' or responses such as: 'Well, it's how you are, you know, what your health is like'. The healers were similarly vague in their responses to my attempts at ascertaining what it was that they were measuring: 'Well, it's their wool, it shows how they are'. The words used by one healer – 'I measured his wool and he was measuring terrible' – suggest that the wool contains or indicates the sufferer's state of illness or wellness.

There are parallels here with orthodox medicine where various methods of measurement of such things as temperature and blood pressure are also employed and patients may be unaware of what is being measured or of its significance. However, in these instances those doing the measuring should (but may not if untrained staff are used) know what is being measured. As with wool measuring these procedures are used to aid the diagnosis and monitoring of disease, but there also may be a therapeutic effect in their performance in that they make patients and measurers feel that something is being done.

There would seem also to be a ritualistic element to medical measurement in terms of the symbolism and mystique of the tools employed, such as the sphygmomanometer and stethoscope, and also the lack of any manifest technological effect. In the above examples from medicine, the measurements fulfil patient expectations that knowledgeable people are investigating their condition and/or monitoring their progress. At the same time, the taking of measurements enables the professionals to feel that they are doing what is required in terms of diagnosing and monitoring sickness. Significantly, the word 'measure' also occurs in the frequently used expressions of 'having the measure' of someone or 'getting the measure of' something, implying gaining essential knowledge and/or control about someone or something.

Given that measurement is both a diagnostic and a healing practice, it may be that the unit of measurement – the length of the wool – is more than just a marking device. As Hand suggests, it may be 'a sort of intermediate agent ... to which the disease is communicated in the process of measurement (Hand 1980: 94). This links in with the concept (frequently referred to in the folk-healing literature) of the transference of illness; that is, the idea that the sufferer needs some sort of intermediate channel through which they may be rid of their illness. Indeed, one healer commented that as he drew on the wool he would 'touch the mind' of the sufferer, suggesting that the wool is a way of connecting with the psyche of the sufferer, and drawing away their illness.

Measuring sometimes also implies containment of a problem. As Hand notes, regarding measurement practices in North America, 'Common to these forms, as well as to certain other kinds of magical measurement for disease, is the notion that the unit of measure, the length marked, or the area circumscribed somehow prevents the ravage of the disease beyond the confines measured' (ibid.: 93). This would suggest that by measuring the sufferer's wool the sickness is perceived as being kept in check in some way; as though, by 'having the measure of it', the healer can keep it under control. This containment notion would tend to fit in with the healers' description of the wool shortening with subsequent measurements – indicating improvement and suggesting that the measurement has stopped the illness getting out of hand.

Reciting 'Special Words'

In addition to the measuring ritual, some healers, while measuring the wool, also recited special, extremely secret, words. I was not witness to the use of these words; those healers that used such words explained to me what they did, but I was not invited to watch. In one of the cases a healer thought he would certainly lose his healing ability if he divulged his words to an outsider. In two instances the words had been actually written down and passed down to the healers from those who had taught them their craft; one of these kept them upstairs in her home, the other in her handbag. These words were apparently biblical in origin and muttered under the healers' breath as they measured. Sufferers were not able to construe what they were; those that heard them at all described them as 'mutterings' and some assumed that they were a prayer.

It seems that these words, if used, are part of the ritual process; that is, they are symbols that are manipulated. It is interesting that sufferers are barely aware of them, suggesting that they are there chiefly for the benefit of the healer, almost a symbolic prop. The fact that those sufferers that heard them interpreted them as being a prayer may again be indicative of their particular cultural frame of reference; that is, their experience of the supernatural is understood within their religious experience.

Type of Wool Used

Two of the healers placed great emphasis on the type of wool, one commenting that it 'had to be pure Welsh wool' and one that it was very important to use the right wool, 'thick Welsh wool, the kind you use for darning socks'. In fact this second healer was finding it so difficult to obtain the right sort of wool that she was considering whether to discontinue the practice. The fact that both healers stressed the importance of the Welsh-ness of the wool is significant in rooting the practice firmly in Welsh culture and tradition. The colour of the wool appears to have been important in the past; Hancock described the use of 'a thread of clean white woollen yarn having a fair twist on it' (Hancock 1873: 328). Whiteness is often symbolically associated with purity and healing. Winstanley and Rose, however, reported the use of crimson wool for the treatment of rheumatism, and commented that 'the colour is probably chosen as being warm, and therefore adverse to the cold disease' (Winstanley and Rose 1926: 173).

Making a Diagnosis

The question of diagnosis or identification of the problem for both sufferer and healer is intriguing in a number of ways. First, as Csordas and Kleinman note, attempting to distinguish between diagnosis and treatment 'reflects our own cultural presuppositions about the nature of healing ... borrowed from clinical practice, [and it] breaks down almost as soon as it is applied in comparative therapeutic systems' (Csordas and Kleinman 1996: 4). Thus, it seems that to insist on such a distinction would be ethnocentric, a biomedical presumption that these two phenomena are always separate. Certainly in the description of the wool measuring, healing is an inherent part of the diagnostic procedure. Moreover, as Helman (2007) notes, diagnosing, or giving a name to a condition, is a form of treatment in a psychological sense inasmuch as it reduces uncertainty and anxiety in patient and family by converting the unknown into the known.

However, although diagnosis and healing are encompassed in the same measuring procedure, the healers did actually separate diagnosis from healing to the extent that they made a point of informing sufferers, or their surrogates, what the wool showed about the state of their health. They attached some importance to diagnosis, especially in terms of differentiating between illness conditions; that is, they regarded it as important that sufferers with conditions other than depression sought appropriate help. One of the healers commented that, 'if they felt ill and the wool wasn't showing anything at all, well, you'd have to tell them to go to the doctor's. But on the other hand if I keep measuring their wool it will help them along'.

Another aspect of diagnosis is that very often this happened prior to consultation in as much as the sufferers or their families may have already self diagnosed 'depression', and hence the need to seek woollen yarn measurement. In these cases, the measuring served to confirm that there was a problem, possibly validating the illness and selection of healer. In addition, the consultation indicated the severity of the illness by the amount of discrepancy in the length of the wool. In some instances the healer made a diagnosis prior to the consultation, based on information about the sufferer that they were privy to from the community or from their observations of the sufferer's appearance. Again, wool measuring confirmed the healer's diagnosis indicating the severity of the illness and providing justification for continued measuring.

A final issue concerning diagnosis is that, as noted earlier, there was no requirement for a face-to-face meeting between healer and patient, although this did happen in many instances requests for healing could be made by the sufferers or on their behalf by surrogates by telephone or letter. Provided the healer had the required information of full name and date of birth the measuring could proceed. This situation is obviously in marked contrast to most other forms of 'alternative' healing where establishing rapport with the client and taking a long personal and illness history is deemed to be of paramount importance; indeed, the efficacy of the treatment usually depends on it. Spending time with clients is often seen to be a particular strength of alternative healers, as opposed to conventional medicine and its much quoted 'six minutes for the patient'. The apparent lack of this in wool measuring is intriguing.

The Shared Meaning of 'Depression'

A prominent theme throughout sociological and anthropological literature is that illness is culturally defined; that is, that social organization and cultural beliefs influence the experience and interpretation of illness (Kleinman 1980; Stacey 1988). Present-day healers employing wool measuring almost always treat what the people in the communities studied – both healers and sufferers – defined as 'depression'. Moreover, for both parties, this depression was firmly situated in terms of its causes and consequences, in the culture of everyday life. In terms of aetiology, depression was seen as a common problem that could befall anyone, arising from the problems of living. The condition frequently, though not always, resulted in sufferers withdrawing from society, in many instances taking to their beds for considerable periods. This understanding of depression resonates with Rubel's notion of 'folk' illnesses, which he explains as 'syndromes from which members of a particular group claim to suffer and for which their culture provides an etiology, diagnosis, preventive measures and regimens of healing' (Rubel 1977: 120).

Depression, as previously noted, tends to be a vague catch-all term describing a state of not feeling emotionally well; it often includes varying degrees of sadness, 'nerves', anxiety and feelings of being unable to cope. This state appears to be brought about by various general problems of everyday life, such as problems in family relationships, financial worries, the after-effects of a debilitating physical illness, and also by bereavement – especially the loss of a partner but also the loss of family and friends. The last category of causative factors is significant in the light of the elderly age of the sufferers in that people in this age group are more likely to be suffering bereavement of family or friends. This is borne out by the interviews in that three of the twelve sufferers described sadness following bereavement; additionally, the healers commented that many of the sufferers or their surrogates identified bereavement as contributing to the sufferer's sadness.

I suggest that what is significant about the causative factors (as perceived by those involved) is the fact that these problems are the stuff of everyday life, and there is no avoiding them. Consequently, the illness deemed to be provoked by these factors is also unavoidable: life's events will provoke sadness, and therefore this illness is less likely to have any blame or stigma attached to it. It was apparent in the interviews with sufferers and healers that depressive illnesses did not carry any stigma or shame; rather, it was something that happened to people at various stages of life and needed to be treated. This was also made explicit in the contrast between biomedical approaches to treatment for depression and wool measuring. Whereas biomedical treatment is firmly committed to keeping the diagnosis of any sort of mental illness confidential, a sufferer's need for wool measuring was discussed without any qualms within the community, and it was not seen as anything to be secretive or ashamed about. A by-product of sufferers' conditions being made public knowledge was that the rest of the community were aware of the need to offer help and support.

After the Measurement

The normal progression of events following measurement is for sufferers to gradually improve. Their progress is monitored, and further healing is given if necessary by continued measuring, usually about three times a day. One of the healers also recommended that, following measurement, sufferers should take one of the following 'tonics', which she learned from the healer who had taught her wool measuring: gin and saffron, whereby one gram of saffron is added to a large bottle of gin and one teaspoon of the concoction is to be taken morning and night; a mixture of egg beaten into a glass of sherry is to be taken daily; a pint of beer stirred with a red hot piece of steel is to be drunk daily.

There are a number of references to prescriptions of potions in addition to wool measuring in the folk literature, as mentioned above. Jones (1930), discussed the hot steel and beer recipe, as well as the use of saffron; and Winstanley and Rose also note that the healer, after measuring their wool, gives clients 'drinks made from herbs' (Winstanley and Rose 1926: 173). It seems likely that the symbolic value of tonics lies in the fact that they are part of local folklore; that is, they are embedded in the community's cultural framework in the same way that wool measuring is.

A number of informants, both sufferers and healers, described the practice of a now deceased healer who tied a piece of wool quite tightly around the sufferer's wrist, which, when it slackened, showed that healing had taken place. This particular healer also used to send a piece of wool through the post with the above described instructions. Similarly, as already mentioned, there are frequent references in the folklore literature to wool being tied around various parts of the body (Hancock 1873; Jones 1930). For instance, Jones noted that 'if the yarn showed the presence of the heart complaint, it was tied round the patient's arm until a cure was accomplished' (1930: 131).

This attachment of the wool to the sufferer's body is very redolent of two frequently occurring themes in folk healing – the use of charms or amulets to protect against illness or misfortune, and the idea of the transference of an illness through some sort of intermediate agent. There are numerous examples in the folk healing literature of people, and indeed animals, being furnished with charms written on leather or paper and worn. It may have been that the actual wearing of woollen threads for a period of time was seen as healing and protective.

The notion of transference is suggested when the thread is actually discarded (for instance when it became slack in the example described above), and the illness is disposed of with it; the thread is then the agent of transference. The concept of transference is illustrated by another example of an informant who was healed of severe hay fever with wool measuring by a now deceased healer. In this case, after measuring, the healer took the thread and threw it in the fire as if to symbolically burn the affliction with it. However, present day wool measurers in this study definitely do not attach the wool to any part of the sufferer's body. It is perplexing that such a substantial change in modus operandi should have occurred in the space of one generation. No one was able to give any explanation for this and due to the small size of the sample group of healers it is not possible to draw any conclusions about this change.

Participants' Understandings of the Process

Not one of the sufferers even attempted to explain how they thought wool measuring worked. Although they would speak at length about other aspects of the encounter, such as how they had felt prior to treatment, the difference the healing had made to them and, very often, the precise time they had started to feel better, it seemed as if the meaning of what had happened was a mystery they thought it better not to question. For example, one sufferer reported, 'I had been feeling so low, then at half-past two [coinciding with the time that he was later informed that wool measuring had taken place], it was as though a heavy cloud had lifted from my head'. He had no explanation for this phenomenon.

It is possible that wool measuring efficacy lies in its incomprehensibility, in that this somehow takes the responsibility away from the sufferer and into the realms of what informants describe as 'magic'. Again, much biomedical healing is also incomprehensible to sufferers. However, one healer was most adamant that the healing was not brought about by magic in any way and she emphasised what she defined as the 'religious nature' of her healing in terms of the necessity of belief in God.

All of the healers expressed a belief that faith was a key element of the process and that sufferers must have faith in the healing practice. In cases where sufferers were unaware that they were being healed, the healers felt that someone must have the faith for them, for instance the person who requested the healing. One healer who felt that he 'touched the mind' of the sufferer through the measurement, commented that although he was unable to say how it worked, he felt that by concentrating on the sufferer's details and making a connection with their mind, the 'cure', as he put it, came from the sufferer's own self. The role of faith may also be seen in relation to the previously discussed organisation of different social networks. That is, in order for individuals to know about wool measuring, and for it to work for them, there needs to be an interlinking of a specific range of cultural connections, such as kinship, chapel membership, language and Welsh identity.

'Feeling Better': The Efficacy of Wool Measuring

In order to evaluate the efficacy of wool measuring as a therapy – that is, whether or not sufferers and their families feel that there is an improvement – it is necessary to identify what sufferers and healers perceive as a successful outcome, as any assessment of success is necessarily subjective. If 'feeling better' is evidence of efficacy, then it appears that wool measuring achieves its goals since all of the sufferers interviewed (and their families if they were present at the interview) said that they felt noticeably better following the measuring. A yardstick of how much better sufferers felt was very often their ability to return to their normal activities, and especially to activities outside the home; that is, back into wider society. Hence people's accounts of improvement were frequently framed in terms what they were able to do and where they were able to go. Thus, an informant describing an improvement in a friend who she had referred for measuring reported: 'In a few days [following measuring] I rang X [the sufferer], and I said. "You feeling better X", and she said "Well, I must be, I'm up the ladder painting"'.

Another sufferer (following measuring) commented: 'I feel like my old self again, I'll go out'. Similarly, one of the healers recounted: 'Another lady, her husband had died, her ninety-year-old mother lived with her, and both of them were unwell. I measured their wool, and she rang to say they had been out for the first time in three months'. And likewise, in the case of a four-year-old who was measured, the proof that she was better was her return to school. It seems that whereas the depressive illness had caused them to withdraw from society, to take to their beds in many cases, the cure had enabled them to return to their usual activities and previous place within their community.

When asked about failure, which appeared to be extremely rare, healers invariably explained it in terms of the original condition being more serious than simple depression. This is exemplified by the following response from a healer: 'Well, I haven't found anyone that I can't heal; they've all said that they're much better. But if there's something else on them that you can't heal, well the only thing that you can do is keep their spirits up, if they're suffering from something else'.

All the healers made it quite clear that they were aware of their limitations; for example, they knew that they could not cure a serious physical illness such as cancer. The above example also illustrates the difficulty in actually evaluating a successful outcome, in that 'feeling better', while not necessarily indicating that they were cured (made free of their illness), especially in biomedical terms, surely indicates success. The person is healed in as much as they no longer feel ill, which is why the wool measuring was sought in the first place.

Conclusion

This chapter has explored the ways in which the culture of particular Welsh-speaking rural communities in mid Wales has influenced the ways in which people experience and understand the condition which they define as 'depression' or *clefyd-y-galon,* which some informants translated as 'sick at heart'. It has been argued that this condition was understood by both sufferers and healers to be situated, in terms of its causation and consequences, in the culture of everyday life. That is, the condition arose from everyday problems of living and was experienced both physically and socially.

The chapter also illustrates the ways in which these communities have developed a repertoire of explanatory frameworks for classifying ambiguous events (such as when people withdraw from society and/or take to their beds) and deciding what legitimately counts as illness. Sufferers in these situations are clearly regarded as being ill and in need of help and support but are channelled by their community towards an alternative healing system that no longer applies to most somatic illness. The cultural construction of depression within these communities illustrates a shared belief system linking members to a wider, historically situated, Welsh culture. For the people of these rural Welsh communities, 'depression' is perceived as a condition arising from the trials of everyday life, recognised by particular behaviour and amenable to treatment by the very ancient practice of wool measuring.

Notes

1. 'Depression' is the term used by respondents in this study to describe their emotional state; it does not necessarily correspond to the medical diagnosis of depression.
2. I use the term 'sufferer' to refer to a person deemed (by themselves or others) to require healing.
3. *Dyn Hysbys* (and the feminine *Dynes Hysbys*) refer to the Welsh version of a 'wise' or 'cunning' man or woman.
4. The words *edau* and *edef* both refer to thread or yarn but reflect different regional dialects.
5. See, e.g., the earlier account from Jones (1930).
6. See Jones (1993) for a discussion of areas heavily influenced by in-migration.

References

Bowie, F. 1993. 'Wales from Within: Conflicting Interpretations of Welsh Identity', in S. Macdonald (ed.) *Inside European Identities*. Oxford: Berg.

Csordas, T.J. and A. Kleinman. 1996. 'The Therapeutic Process', in T.M. Johnson and C.F. Sargent (eds), *Medical Anthropology*. Westport, CT: Greenwood Press.

Davies, C.A. 1999. *Reflexive Ethnography: A Guide to Researching Selves and Others*. London: Routledge.

Davies, J.C. 1911. *Folklore of West and Mid Wales*. Aberystwyth: Welsh Gazette Offices.

Davies, W.L. 1938. 'The Conjuror in Montgomeryshire', *Montgomeryshire Collections* 45: 158–70.

Evans, R.M. 1937. 'Folklore and Customs in Cardiganshire', *Transactions of the Cardiganshire Antiquarian Society* 12: 52–58.

Good, B. 1977. 'The Heart of What's the Matter: The Semantics of Illness in Iran', *Culture, Medicine and Psychiatry* 1: 25–58.

Hancock, T.W. 1873. 'Llanrhaiadr-yn-Mochnant, its Parochial History and Antiquities', *Montgomeryshire Collections* 6: 319–40.

Hand, W.T. 1980. *Magical Medicine*. Berkeley: University of California Press.

Helman, C.G. 2007. *Culture, Health and Illness*, 5th edn. Oxford: Butterworth-Heinemann.

Jones, N. 1993. *Living in Rural Wales*. Llandysul: Gomer.

Jones, T.G. 1930. *Welsh Folk Lore and Folk Custom*. London: Methuen.

Kleinman, A. 1980. *Patients and Healers in the Context of Culture*. Berkeley: University of California Press.

———. 1986 'Concepts and a Model for the Comparison of Medical Systems as Cultural Systems', in C. Currer and M. Stacey (eds), *Concepts of Health, Illness and Disease: A Comparative Perspective*. Oxford: Berg.

Nordland, O. 1961. 'The Street of the Wise Women: A Contribution to the Sociology of Folk-medicine' *Arv: Journal of Scandinavian Folklore*, 18-19: 105–116.

Owen, E. 1887. *Welsh Folklore*. Wakefield: E.P. Publishing.

Peate, I. 1924. 'The Dyfi Basin: Its People, Antiquities, Dialects, Folklore and Place Names', M.A. thesis. Aberystwyth: University of Wales.

Prior, L. 2003. *Using Documents in Social Research*. London: Sage.

Rubel, A.J. 1977 'The Epidemiology of a Folk Illness', in D. Landy (ed.) *Culture, Disease and Healing: Studies in Medical Anthropology*. New York: Macmillan.

Scott, J. 1990. *A Matter of Record*. Cambridge: Polity Press.

Spradley, J.P. 1980. *Participant Observation*. New York: Holt, Rinehart and Winston.

St Clair, S. 1971. *Folklore of the Ulster People*. Cork: Mercier Press.

Stacey, M. 1988. *The Sociology of Health and Healing*. London: Routledge.

Thomas, K. 1971. *Religion and the Decline of Magic*. Letchworth: Garden City Press.

Thorndike, L. 1923. *A History of Magic and Experimental Science, Volume I*. New York: Columbia University Press.

Williams, R. 1888. 'History of the Parish of Llanbrynmair' *Montgomeryshire Collections* 22: 35–328.

Westropp, T.J. 1911. 'A Folklore Survey of County Clare', *Folklore* 22: 49–60.

Winstanley, L. and H.J. Rose. 1926. 'Scraps of Welsh Folklore, I' *Folklore* 38: 154–74.

Chapter 5

A General Practice, A Country Practice: The Cure, the Charm and Informal Healing in Northern Ireland

Ronnie Moore

This chapter discusses findings from ethnographic research conducted in 1995/6 in two small rural towns in Northern Ireland, Ballymacross and Hunterstown, the former predominantly Roman Catholic and the latter predominantly Protestant.[1] The discussion pays particular attention to the role of informal healing, handed down between generations as an oral tradition, and how this is juxtaposed and integrated into general healthcare practices in both communities. It focuses on a specifically Irish form of folk healing referred to locally as 'the 'cure' or 'the charm', and looks at how this is embedded in local belief systems, how it impacts on the social and economic structure of both communities, and how this is seen to operate – that is, how and by what mechanisms the gift of the cure/charm is inherited or transferred.

The discussion highlights the interface between local people and formal health care systems; how health belief systems impact on such issues as service provision and the uptake of services; and the duties and limitations of the role of general practitioner (GPs) other health care professionals and local chemists. It also considers information needs and information exchange.

Background to the Research

The research project on which this chapter draws came about as a result of a government focus on targeting health and social needs which arose from a response to a Department of Health White Paper and the locally applied interpretations of this (see, respectively, DoH 1992; DHSS 1995). Northern Ireland has been unique in integrating health and social care structures at Department and Health Authority levels. The central thrust of the research sought to assess health and related needs in each community and a major priority was the interpretation and experiences of health and illness by local people. Several quantitative studies had been completed prior to this investigation and although they revealed much, they also pointed up considerable limitations when it came to looking at nuanced health beliefs and behaviour (Stringer 1990; Robson, Bradford and Deas 1994).[2]

This study sought an emic perspective and looked at how local people viewed health, illness and associated service provision, and how these views affected the everyday lives of individuals and those of their family and community. It was concerned with self-reported health, on factors influencing health status and health chances, health service provision and take up, perceptions of health care delivery, and how local people prioritised health needs.

The actual fieldwork phase lasted for a period of four months in each community and these were studied consecutively. The Provisional Irish Republican Army (IRA) and Protestant paramilitary ceasefires of 1995/6 helped facilitate the fieldworker's entry into these communities. A detailed account of the rationale for the study, details on the methodology employed, including population size, location and choice of towns, is presented elsewhere (Moore et al. 1996). The key findings were produced as two separate reports for the Department of Health and Social Services (DHSS) of Northern Ireland, and in several published papers. These emphasised multiple and interrelated factors as determinants of health, health behaviour and health capital (Moore et al. 1997a, 1997b; Moore 2007). A significant finding from the fieldwork was the belief in, and local commitment to, folk healing as an integral part of a broad canopy of health belief and health resources. Local people utilised health-belief models that paradoxically straddled both formal (scientific) and lay (superstitious) accounts of health and illness with relative ease. This was the case for both towns.

Ballymacross and Hunterstown are small, encapsulated market towns in Northern Ireland. The local economy is mostly agricultural. Sheep, cattle and dairy farming are important sources of income, as are family run businesses, some small, some large. Smallholdings are more common in Ballymacross than in Hunterstown, where farms tend to be larger. Northern Ireland is highly segregated with a majority of people preferring to live among 'their own'. There was a general tendency to marry within the locality and remain geographically close to kin. Marriage was traditionally endogamous and mixed marriages between Protestants and Catholics tended to be infrequent. The lack of intermarriage restricted Protestant and Catholic interaction at the personal level.

The historical background to civil unrest in Northern Ireland points to religious affiliation as the basis of physical, social and ethnic divisions. Northern Ireland is commonly portrayed as a clash of two cultures, two religions – Catholic and Protestant – and two national identities, British and Irish. Religion is an important marker for national, regional and local identity (see Geertz 1966). The idea of nationhood expresses awareness and sentiments of belonging. For Geertz, it is representative of a network of extended kinship or common ancestors. Others, such as Anderson (1983), suggest that even when this is not actually the case, the idea or 'imagination' of what makes up a nation or a community has important consequences. Anderson's constructionist approach defines a more fluid account of 'the nation' and the idea of nationalism (also including fictive notions of common ancestry) within the context of culture. For Anderson these crucially represent important political communities and continuities.

In this sense, religion is representative of a cultural system, and engenders a sense of belonging to a real or 'imagined community'. It therefore influences such things as social organisation, identity, physical and mental boundaries, as well as a sense of belonging, language and expression, a sense of security, neighbourliness and co-operation, and also conflict (Moore 2004). Religion-as-culture is the basis of the two major ethno-religious identities in Northern Ireland, Protestants and Roman Catholics.

As a consequence, many communities in Northern Ireland live separate and encapsulated lives. More than 60 per cent of the population prefer to live in areas where more than 80 per cent of their neighbours share their religion (O'Reilly and Stevenson 1998). Almost 50 per cent of Protestants said they would rather live in an all-Protestant area, and 43 per cent said they would not allow a member of their family to marry a Catholic (Murtagh 1996: 31). Contacts outside the local community are therefore limited. This has consequences in terms of stereotyping, world-view, political attitudes and the strength of boundaries. The expression of boundaries is strongest in working-class areas, both urban and rural. 'Networks that divide are largely based on pragmatic and uniplex relationships.... Multiplex ties are more likely in the case of the professional classes' (Moore and Sanders 1996: 135). These historical beliefs and practices continue ethno-religious differentiation. They are (for many) an important basis for division. On the one hand, Catholics and Protestants in Northern Ireland share a common culture (see Larsen 1982; Moore and Sanders 1996), yet they are separated on the basis of religious affiliation and express different habitus (Lundy and McGovern 2007; Moore 2007).

Historically, Northern Ireland had a highly developed industrial base. The early development of capitalism extends back to Huguenot lace-making in the late 1600s and the production of linen, while heavy engineering, shipbuilding and leadership in commerce and industry put Northern Ireland on a world stage. However, the province began to experience a process of deindustrialisation in the early twentieth century, and in the period immediately after the Second World War the industrial base was in irreversible decline with mass redundancies in linen manufacturing and shipbuilding (Howe 1990). Unemployment became a structural feature of the economy, particularly in the wake of the oil crises of the 1970s. For some, employment opportunities lay elsewhere and it was not unusual for individual family members from Ballymacross and Hunterstown to work and live abroad. Historically, this has meant migration to the U.S.A. and mainland Britain, but in recent times the economic upturn in the Republic of Ireland offered new employment prospects.

Ballymacross was perceived (by insiders and outsiders) as a Catholic town, although some Protestants lived in the surrounding locality. It developed in the middle of the eighteenth century as a market town and centre for livestock and linen. Nestled in a mountainous picturesque landscape, where the land tended to be poor, the main source of agriculture was sheep farming, although some dairy farming was also practiced. Catholicism was an important feature in Ballymacross, defining spiritual, ethnic and political identity, and was a major feature of social and community life. The Catholic Church was a key institution, and it not only provided moral guidance but was also important in terms of local community surveillance and in regulating social behaviour. There was no police station in the town. This role fell to the local priests and to significant individuals such as local community leaders. The Church was actively engaged in many aspects of social life and social activities, and emphasised community integration and social and religious solidarity. Church clubs and the Gaelic Athletic Association (GAA) reinforced links within the parish, signifying Ballymacross as a separate and distinct community from other (including Catholic) towns and town lands. The dominance of the GAA also meant that other outlooks such as political and cultural interests tended to be shared.

There were no general practitioners (GPs) based in Ballymacross. The nearest health centre was two miles away in a neighbouring, predominantly Protestant town. Multiple layers of health resources were evident. Strong extended family networks and neighbourliness operated as a crucial system of informal welfare and health capital,[3] while formal healthcare offered a professional service. Also, the local pharmacist was a central figure and important point of contact with the formal healthcare system, and they were a significant resource for people in Ballymacross, partly because of the absence of a local GP. Not only was he trained in pharmacy, but he was also indigenous to the town, had deep local, cultural and personal knowledge of his neighbours and clients, and could communicate with people in an informal and discreet manner. He was a respected figure who also owned and ran one of the six public houses in the town and saw people on a daily basis outside his role as a pharmacist. His advice and assistance could be sought, both day and night, and in many respects he took on the role of the doctor.

Hunterstown was first settled in the early seventeenth century by Scots and English through the plantation of Ireland,[4] and parish records indicate a wide range of developing occupations. Becoming a thriving town during the industrial revolution, farms here tended to be bigger than in Ballymacross and Hunterstown developed into a major livestock centre, this being an important part of the local economy. The social structure of Hunterstown was also more complex than that of Ballymacross. Families were similarly close-knit but there was a high degree of social segmentation, with social-class cleavages more in evidence. Religious denomination was also a source of social differentiation. There were various Protestant denominations present, as well as smaller sects, and Roman Catholics living in or around the town accounted for less than 20 percent of the overall population (Moore et al. 1997a). In addition, there were those who regarded themselves as not being particularly religious – known locally as the 'good living' – but who identified themselves as being culturally Protestant. Though the Orange Order was born in the local area,[5] social and political unity was often expressed only periodically, such as on ceremonial occasions or at times of political uncertainty or political violence, when both communities polarised.[6] Unlike Ballymacross, Hunterstown had a health centre. The role of the pharmacist differed from that of Ballymacross in that it was a small part of healthcare provision in the town and not a principal feature of it.

When comparing the two communities, there were a number of notable features. Ballymacross typified many rural Catholic towns in Northern Ireland. The Church was a major unifying feature in terms of local and national identity. Ballymacross was characterised by a more homogeneous and stable social and political ethos and identity. Hunterstown, meanwhile, was also typical of many rural Protestant towns in Northern Ireland. In contrast to Ballymacross, it was less egalitarian. It emphasised historical denominational divisions as well as fundamentalist factions and those who were not particularly religious. For Protestants in Hunterstown, there was no single overarching, unified Church or moral authority.

In Ballymacross, religious observance was a major community expectation and social integration was culturally expected. Local people felt compelled by local mores and rules to conform to local beliefs, behaviour and social and political outlook. As a social worker from Ballymacross commented, 'I work by different rules when I'm here'. As Weber noted, Protestantism historically emphasised religious freedom and personal piety and stressed autonomy and destiny. Indeed, this was generally regarded as a necessary precondition for the vigour of rational capitalist development (Hamilton 2001). Protestantism subjectified and emphasised asceticism and personal success for salvation. Weber's concept of 'inner loneliness' was thought to typify Calvinist doctrine and lifestyle. In Hunterstown, social atomisation and individualism featured more strongly than in Ballymacross.

The Catholic community was seen as supporting a unified Catholic ethos and identity with the strict involvement of religion and the Church, while the Protestant community reflected not only historical denominational divisions but also more recent factions in the form of new (inspirational) Protestantism. Protestantism was not supportive of a cohesive collective identity on a day-to-day basis; rather, the opposite was true (Moore 2004). Given the ethnographic profile of each of these towns, one might reasonably hypothesise that since the historical and ethno-religious bases of social division have been (and remain) so profound, then health beliefs, health behaviours and health outlooks might also differ.

Ethno-religious identity provide the basis for such a view. The communities differed in the degree and scope of social capital potential. Catholics were seen to be more closely aligned to a religious ethos and the notion of the spiritual and the supernatural. We could, therefore, argue (as many classic sociological texts do) that, conversely, Protestants display more rationality, and thus reject supernatural and superstitious beliefs such as folk healing, and instead rely more on formal medicine. This is a plausible argument, with supporting evidence from Graham's study of Mexican-Americans. Graham notes that, 'The great majority of those who accept to one degree or another the folk medical system are Catholic, and for them Catholicism is as much a way of life as it is a religion' (Graham 1985: 169). However, Graham also points out that, 'if a person is male, Protestant, well educated, fairly young, and has grown up in a middle-class family … [h]e will probably rely exclusively on institutionalised medicine' (ibid.: 181).

My own research, however, argues that while Protestant and Catholic communities in Northern Ireland each displayed a different habitus, they also emphasised common lay health beliefs, health knowledge and health strategies. Belief in the supernatural and folk healing practices was central to this and was embedded in Hunterstown at least to the same degree as in Ballymacross. Notable exemplars of the continuance and pervasiveness of supernatural belief in this community lie in Protestant lay clergy and fundamentalist Churches that typify the belief in the actual embodiment of God and the Devil. Speaking in tongues, the laying on of hands, the belief in miracle cures and the casting-off of demons are not foreign to this tradition. In more recent times this has been internationalised by prominent preachers from Billy Graham to current televangelists such as Benny Hinn.

The Cure, the Charm and Informal Healing in Northern Ireland

In both Northern Ireland and Southern Ireland there are individuals who are identified as having special mystical healing properties, and people in Ballymacross and Hunterstown referred to a people from the parish who had the gift of healing. Strongly embedded in the local culture of both towns was the belief in 'the cure' or 'the charm', terms which were interchangeable.[7] People in both communities were aware that, if needs be, they could readily access folk healers and many had gone for, or had had a relative go for, a cure/charm. Cures could be obtained for various conditions or for multiple health problems. These were mostly, but not always for minor complaints, such as skin conditions – such as warts, ringworm or shingles – but people also sought cures for the most serious conditions, including cancers. This might be as an initial or last resort, but was more often done in conjunction with other formal healthcare treatment. It all depended on the nature of the condition.

Cures, curing, and healing were not casually talked about yet it was well understood that the cure/charm was a public, or community, resource. Information on cures and charms was not normally volunteered but was usually spoken of only at times of crisis, often introduced by a family member or close friend in a personal and private context. Knowledge pertaining to cures was private and the potency of the practice was thought to depend upon belief and a commitment to respecting and maintaining these unspoken rules. The act of recommending a cure/charm was interpreted as an act of neighbourliness in both towns, and the process bound local people together in a special locally understood way.

As information on cures/charms emerged during fieldwork, the approach was to minimise a priori assumptions and not to seek out available literature on folk healing practices until after data was collected. The School of Irish, Celtic Studies, Irish Folklore and Linguistics at University College Dublin holds the Irish archive of accounts of charms and remedies, and there is a limited, although established, literature on folk healing in Northern Ireland. Publications on folk healing range from popularised accounts (see Lady Wilde cited in Barry 1990 [original nd]) to more recent attempts at scholarly explanations of Irish cures and folk medicine (Logan 1981). Fleetwood (1983[1951]), for example, in the opening of his history of medicine in Ireland, discusses folk medicine, and Cox (Chapter 2, this volume) reviews important literature with respect to the Republic of Ireland. We may add to this Murphy and Kelleher (1995) and, specific to Northern Ireland, the very useful accounts presented by Buckley (1980). Roch (1981), a medical practitioner herself, also provides a useful summary of the literature. In addition, there are more recent works of MacFarlane (1998) and MacFarlane and Ginnety (2001).

Many people interviewed had themselves chosen to seek a cure/charm for an illness or condition at some point. The oral tradition ensured continuity and this hinged on personal faith, childhood socialisation, general community belief, personal experience and hearsay. The gift of the cure may be obtained in a number of well-defined and locally sanctioned ways. The folk healer needs to be identified and locally recognised as a curer and the rules defining this are clear to all in the community.

The cure was assigned to the healer on the bases of inheritance, birthright, or via some other special circumstances. Local people said that the gift of the cure was normally passed from mother to son or father to daughter. In some instances this was very specific. For example, it was commonly believed that someone who was born after the death of their father automatically assumed the cure for oral thrush or 'badmouth' irrespective of whether the father had the cure. Marrying someone with the same surname was believed to bestow a gift of the cure. The seventh son was believed to have the ability to cure, and the most potent healing power was believed to be held by the seventh son of a seventh son. However, as Buckley noted, there is an essential difference between forms of divine healing, which claim specific reference to God and often have an international dimension, and the cure/charm, which is peculiarly Irish:

> 'Divine healing', as many of its practitioners insist on calling it, or 'faith healing' as it is popularly known, is closely related to the cure, and is well known in Ulster, though fewer people practice it (Buckley 1980: 26). The latter, ... is defined by clearly defined cultural rules which admit few variations, the divine healer either decides himself that he should practice healing or else he receives a pressing invitation from God himself. (ibid: 26)

Unlike divine healers, the person with the cure is not motivated by the desire to become a healer nor do they wish to prove, nor seek to make any claims for, efficacy. Also, the practical act of curing was said to vary. It might include combinations of actions, and could involve the laying of hands on affected parts of the body, prayers or incantations, the use of sticks or smoking sticks and/or specially prepared substances or powders, or acts unseen. Some (particularly those who had immigrated or worked abroad) believed that cures could be obtained over the phone, while others in the local community thought this was not the best method to affect a cure: 'For the ringworm, he just used a burning stick and held it over the area. I'm sure he said something, but I can't remember what it was' (Wendy, Hunterstown).

Folk healers did not choose to have the gift. It was bestowed on them and they chose to keep it and to use it or not. Some were reluctant practitioners driven by a sense of expectancy and social obligation rather than by personal choice, feeling duty bound because of community expectation to act as healers. Curers did not seek, or necessarily accept, monetary payment for their services, though they might (but not always) accept payment in kind.

> I just went to her three times and then the last time I brought her out fruit and teabags. (Angie, Hunterstown)
>
> I would believe in them. There is a woman down in Ballymacross now and she has the cure for haemorrhage, she just rubs her hands. She cured me of a sprain years ago. She doesn't charge anything, you know. She doesn't take any money off you. Then there is Dan D–. Everybody goes to him. (Nan, Ballymacross)

There were local sceptics in both communities, but a broad range of people from varied social backgrounds talked about getting the cure or believing in the power of the cure.

> I have been down that road myself. I'm prepared to do anything at any stage. I would decry them normally, but my youngster had whooping cough a couple of years ago and I beat my way down to K–. It was just horrendous. This was January, and the child was just absolutely horrendous, and I had got to the stage where I had gone to the doctor and then somebody said you need a charm, and I said, 'Point me in the direction of it', and we went down. It was quite funny but I didn t care because she was so fed up and so upset ... You don't think you need them until the time comes, then all the ideas of religion, and your teaching goes by the wayside, because if you see a child sick you would do anything. (Mrs Wilson, Hunterstown)

Teachers, social workers, health professionals, business people as well as ordinary people had gone for, or believed in the cure/charm.

> Well I think it is good if you have the faith [in the cure]. Yes, I have it. My son hurt himself playing football one night at the BB [Boys Brigade] and he was on crutches. He couldn't put his foot down and his grandpa phoned and said about this woman [who] done it and my husband ran him out [i.e. took him to her] and she worked at him for a while. And then she says, 'You can put your crutches away', and he said 'Oh, but I can't put my foot down', and he came home to the house again walking with no crutches ... I don't know what she did now. (Angie, Hunterstown)
>
> I had went [sic] for a charm when I had Andrew for postnatal depression and you were given something to take home ... At that time when you are going through postnatal depression you are dragged along to them, but you are at a point where you would do anything. (Mrs Ray, Ballymacross)

Also, children were at some point taken (usually by their mothers) to recognised healers as part of a socialisation process.

> My mother took me for a cure. I had the shingles one time and she packed me off to this woman. But I'm not sure if it works (Sally, Hunterstown)
>
> I have tried the cure. I went once with my daughter. I thought she had a colic. I went out there thinking, 'I ll try it anyway'. (Sally, Hunterstown)

Several informants also recounted personal discomfort when they were taken as children to a specific healer:

> There was somebody doing a dubious cure. A gentleman who was touching people inappropriately as part of a cure. (Jan, Ballymacross)

The issue was raised with the relevant social services who indicated that they had been aware that this might be a problem, but there had been no officially reported complaints.

The point about the cure is that it is tied to more pagan cosmological ideas of health involving magical and supernatural beliefs, and not necessarily tied to religion or religiosity per se. It is localised, organic, informal healing. While it often did not explain ill health, it pragmatically acted as an alternative therapeutic resource and as a corrective to the limitations of formal medicine. It dealt with specific cases and ailments where formal medicine was uninterested, was deemed to have failed, or was not trusted.

> We went to B–, the two girls had ringworm … It went away very quickly on one, but it took a wee bit longer on the other. We had gone to the doctor but it didn't make any difference. He gave me some sort of anti-fungal cream to put on it. He said it would take care of it, but it didn't. It just got worse. (Wendy, Hunterstown)

Folk healing was integrated into general health care practices in both communities. Also, the cure/charm is as much social as it is magical. The individual with the cure submits to community expectation to fulfil a function as part of their daily life as a healer. In addition (evident particularly in Ballymacross), belief in the cure also acted as a potent binding force for local people. Community life in Northern Ireland has been described as having a strong sense of neighbourliness, community obligation and modesty (Harris 1972). There is also the community expectation of assisting neighbours, particularly if a person becomes ill or in times of personal or family crisis. Recommending a cure therefore was seen as a neighbourly gesture. Many local people thought that healing worked for specific conditions.

Belief in the cure was not necessarily tied to spiritual belief. Those who have the cure, as Buckley notes, 'have no claim to extraordinary religious belief, still less, extraordinary virtue' (Buckley 1980: 31). Healers may have a spiritual faith or may not. The Catholic Church appeared fairly ambivalent about curers. Officially they did not sanction folk healing. Yet it was known in Ballymacross that some Catholic priests (past and present) were also said to have the ability to cure. On the whole, local priests were said to be sympathetic. However, the cosmological beliefs of local people also included aspects of the supernatural that lay outside the strict doctrine of the Church, and folk healing was set aside from other forms of religious supernatural belief. In Protestant Hunterstown, the social structure was more visibly segmented on the bases of social class and denomination, including various evangelical groups. The 'good living' and many who did not express a religious commitment believed in cures.

Health Professional Responses to the Cure/Charm.

Health professionals were not only aware of folk healing but had factored it into their working practice. In other words, although cures were not openly spoken about there was tacit acceptance by local GPs and other healthcare professionals that folk healing was an important aspect of life in these communities. Many health professionals also recognised, in a very practical sense, the valuable presence of people able to administer the cure/charm. Various ailments, most certainly many minor ailments, were treated elsewhere away from the surgery. To this extent, folk healing was viewed by doctors as taking pressure off over-burdened practices.

One GP interviewed said he believed in the cure/charm, while some GPs said they recognised that cures had a therapeutic value. Others were sympathetic, but stopped short of openly supporting the practice. Even sceptical GPs accepted local healing as 'generally harmless' or even beneficial. While one GP interviewed was hostile to folk healing, another said he had referred patients to a local healer: 'They can use them if they want to – they sometimes work'. One local, newly appointed, young GP thought that, 'I used to think they were wee men with a crocked finger who would cure your warts. It is surprising to me the people who are into this. Some of these people are the most sensible cosmopolitan persons you could get'. But this GP was keen to point out his concern about people with serious conditions who had not sought medical help, and said that their deaths could have been avoided if they had consulted a doctor earlier. He recounted an instance where a patient sought a cure rather than medical advice and therefore presented very late with fatal consequences.

Health professionals were acutely aware of local culture beliefs and practices. It was felt that to speak out publicly against cures would mean risking their local reputation and credibility within the community, and yet to acknowledge folk medicine might leave one open to ridicule from peers since it was deemed to have the capacity to undermine the very principles of biomedical training and scientific knowledge. However, GPs interviewed took a pragmatic approach to this. They recognised that biomedical efficacy and their own practice also rested on the acceptance of local cultural ideas about health. In other words, even sceptical GPs were aware that they must work alongside traditional health beliefs and practices. Buchan noted similar concerns in the writings of the physician David Rorie, who lived among ordinary people in rural Scotland and who documented folk practices there in the early twentieth century: 'physicians cannot assume uncritical or passive compliance with their wishes in communities maintaining strong traditional beliefs and a healthy disrespect for scientific authority' (Buchan 1994).[8]

Also, many local professionals interviewed, including health professionals, said they believed in the power of the cure. Several community nurses and health visitors admitted to using traditional healers for ailments themselves, for relatives and for animals: 'We have had animals that have been dehorned and started to bleed and my husband has gone and got the charm and when they came home they stopped bleeding' (Helen, retired nurse manager).

One senior community nurse told of how she had witnessed the cure working on an elderly man who had shingles:

> I have an open mind on charms because I have seen them work both in my professional capacity and in our private life ... I remember once the doctor sending me to an old man who lived more or less like a hermit in an old shack and the doctor said to me, 'You may go down and do the best you can, for that man has shingles; and just get the clothes off him – I don't think they have been off him for many years – and treat him with Gentian Violet'. So on my way home that evening I called and really I never saw anything like it in my whole professional career. And I managed to get the clothes off him and treated him. He says, 'Will you quit worrying nurse, I'm going for the charm tonight'. And I said to myself, 'Oh, does he think he is going to get rid of this in a day or two'. But quite honestly, within a week he was completely cured and I couldn't see it in a month. (Madge, community nurse)

When asked to explain how this could happen, she said she couldn't: 'It was the cure. It simply worked'. Some health visitors also routinely incorporated traditional healing into their own practice:

> I think psychologically, it can do the mums more good. And as long as it doesn't interfere with other treatment, and the child is not getting anything that's going to do any harm. I would sort of say, 'What is it – what cure are you using?' I would sort of investigate that ... I always like to know, 'cause sometimes with colic they could boil milk and could put bits and pieces in it, but normally only take a teaspoon[ful]. I would routinely do that just to see, 'cause you never know what's been recommended. (Kate, Health visitor)

Pharmacists in Ballymacross and Hunterstown firmly expressed their belief in the power of the cure. A chemist (in another town) was also known to have the gift: 'Some chemists had the charm. L–'s chemist in P–. It's very good now. He does it as a sideline. It's actually a charm' (Mrs Frew, Hunterstown).

What was significant was the similarity in terms of the extent of folk knowledge and folk practice in these two encapsulated, religiously segregated, suspicious and defensive rural communities. Folk healing was crucially important in both towns. The reason why folk healing knowledge and practices were common and consistent in Catholic Ballymacross and Protestant Hunterstown was at least in part due to local economics and animal husbandry. In this sense, folk healing had historically impacted on the social and economic structure of both communities.

Local farmers would routinely get cures/charm for their animals. This was not just for bleeding cow horns, but also extended to cures that affected lamb, calf and foal survival. Just as women might be said to be the managers of health in the informal setting, and in the health centre might casually exchange information on health issues pertaining to their family, a similar process of information exchange and consultation regularly took place at the local cattle market where Catholic and Protestant farmers (or their representatives) would be present. Folk healers might also be present: 'Every mart you would go to he [D–] was busy with the sheep' (Wendy, Hunterstown).

The historical connection between cures for animals and humans is a close one. For example, Logan discusses the link with organic inoculation and Jenner's later, scientifically proclaimed link in 1798. The pus from a mild form of smallpox was considered a traditional means to infect and cure healthy individuals. In the case of vaccination, the cowpox virus (closely related to smallpox), is now routinely used with effect. This was considered to be a safer practice and had the desired affect. Although inoculation with smallpox was made illegal in 1840, Logan points to documented cases suggesting its continued usage: 'It was believed that the protection against smallpox given by the doctors' vaccination only lasted for seven years but the protection given by the Donleavy's inoculation lasted for life' (Logan 1981:6).

The cure/charm may also be viewed as an important social transaction in that those who seek or offer cures are reaffirming their commitment to local cultural beliefs and customs regarding health practices. The act of willingly going for a cure/charm or recommending one, while not necessarily taken as proof positive of personal acceptance of the power of the cure, demonstrated an important social and community influence on individuals. This has a magical, religious and moral imperative (even if the cures were needed for animals).

The very foundation of society is rooted upon the relationship between the individual and the group, and the group and the individual.[9] Folk healing is also part of a wider pattern of regulation in terms of individual behaviour. It is concerned with the group feelings of dependence, consolidation, maintenance, solidarity and unity (Durkheim 1915). In this regard, curers are the servitors of society, submissive to the rules of local culture and to wider social forces. It was known that one young man who lived near Ballymacross had the gift of the cure. He had not wished to have it and was away for most of the week attending his university course in Belfast. However, on his return at the weekends he was expected to be available if needed.

The Wider Significance of the Cure/Charm

The cure/charm assumed a central importance in both communities, and health professionals did not only take cognisance of folk healing, but the practice overlapped with formal medicine. Both healthcare systems provided a range of health services that each community knew about and drew upon. In this sense, the relationship between folk medicine and formal medicine was integrated and symbiotic. Formal medicine as a single entity would practice with a greater degree of difficulty in these communities, and both local people and healthcare professionals made this clear. While local GPs were unlikely to state this publicly, many privately believed it. Equally, those with the cure/charm did not seek to usurp the position of doctors. How both modalities were utilised often depended upon illness severity and perceived optimum treatment (from what was deemed the most appropriate system) for that condition. Local people did not simply blindly follow locally derived health knowledge either. Expectations were generally modest and people were well aware of the limitations of folk medicine, just as they were with formal medicine. Folk medicine often filled the gaps, and treated the conditions that formal medicine neglected, misunderstood and/or misdiagnosed.

Rather than repudiate formal medicine, healers offered an alternative to biomedical explanations of illness. Local people understood biomedicine to be devoid of the possibility of other, non-scientific or as yet undiscovered explanations. The constant re-examination of ideas and practices in light of new knowledge, what Giddens (1990) refers to as the 'reflexive implementation of knowledge', is constrained within a training regimen that follows a narrowly prescribed scientific paradigm. Cures, because they lie outside this paradigm, are likely to be medically reframed and explained as placebo effects (if they work) or mumbo-jumbo if it is not proven that they work.

As the above vignettes illustrate, when faced with the boundaries of formal medicine (whether these were with regard to efficacy, communication difficulties, mismatch of expectations, or a clash of health beliefs), there was recourse to folk medicine and this was recognised as an important resource. Local people in both towns also recognised that traditional folk practices by virtue of their survival (and to this degree they were understood to be tested and proven) had been affecting cures long before formal medicine and 'expert systems' had established themselves. This was long established practice based on evidence. Because they were organic, stemming from community ideas and values, they were trusted,[10] whereas modern medicine was treated with suspicion and perceived to be both fallible and harmful.

In recent times the issues of personal risk and public perceptions of risk, trust and scepticism has become a commanding feature in the social-science literature. Expert systems such as biomedicine require trust, yet this research indicates that such trust is conditional. Lay knowledge also calculates risk and takes a pragmatic attitude to expert systems. Landy (1974) illustrates interaction between both different treatment systems, whereby people make choices as to which they use: scientific or folk medicine. Landy refers to this as 'folk pragmatism'.

In Ballymacross and Hunterstown, failures and shortcomings in formal medicine were often recounted, while folk healing (even if it was not witnessed first hand) was remembered for its cures. Formal medicine was said to be remote, increasingly bourgeois, and personally arrogant. There was an acute awareness of social-class distinctions and the feeling that self-aggrandisement and money was a major motivator for those going into the medical profession: 'What I think about the younger doctors is that they are very money orientated' (Mary, Ballymacross). This is in marked contrast to historical descriptions of medical 'men' as being middle class with an apparent aloofness from the struggle of gaining an income (Lawrence 1985),[11] an aloofness that was once deemed an important ingredient in the making of a good physician. The rise of professional medicine, however, changed the nature of the relationship between doctors and their patients. Historically, class-based gentlemen physicians administered to gentlemen (and women). The status shift within medicine involved a move from individual gentlemen physicians to a legally sanctioned and unified profession that was sanctioned by a core body of knowledge and recognised educational institutions and licensing institutions (ibid.) With this came the shift from the isolated family physician – with detailed local knowledge embedded in the community and in its local culture, whose role lay beyond offering a clinical service – towards the new pillars of medical modernity: the laboratory, the medical school and the hospital.

The shift of focus from 'person' to 'condition' and 'disease mechanisms' influenced the style of consultation, and the rise in ultra-scientifically trained doctors, as Bynum and Porter (1993:783–800) note, has led to a crisis of trust in late-modern society and has been at the centre of much sociological inquiry into the nature of the doctor–patient relationship. The resultant alienation of patients from doctors may be directly measured against the growing trend toward a return to earlier healthcare traditions such as alternative medicine and plural health modes, and in the rising numbers of malpractice suits (Lawrence 1985). 'In the United Kingdom: in 1981, alternative practitioners were twenty seven per cent as numerous as the total number of general practitioners; the numbers of acupuncturists doubled between 1978 and 1981; and the consultation of such non orthodox practitioners increased by 4 per cent from 1981 to 1985' (Bynum and Porter 1993: 795). The subjective interpretation of symptoms and signs became less valid medical data as the focus moved towards the notionally 'objective' (and quantifiable) findings of diagnostic technology (see Bynum and Porter 1993:783–800). The belief that physicians now must understand the scientific mechanisms underlying the drugs prescribed influenced the course and emphasis of medical training. However, 'This apparently sensible rationale ignored the realities that, first, it is not at all necessary to understand basic metabolic pathways in order to prescribe successfully; and second, most doctors forget this information anyway after they leave medical school' (Bynum and Porter 1993: 793). The latter point is now highlighted in the development of new Problem-based Learning (PBL) teaching strategies in modern medical schools, designed to help physicians retain information.

Increasingly, modern scientific medicine has been accompanied, as historians and physicians have warned, by a growing dissatisfaction with medical care (Porter 2000; Helman 2007). Mary's point about money-oriented contemporary doctors is illustrative of this dissatisfaction, and her perception was that of the designer-suited bejeweled physician who, although they might be competently grounded in biological and scientific knowledge, lacked a complete understanding of health. Physicians and the medical establishment consistently emphasise science in medicine, believing that what cannot be scientifically explained is unimportant. Worse, high status and high salaries has increased the cultural gap between physicians and the public they serve even further and has helped retain disaffection and disillusionment with biomedicine.[12] Despite this, antagonisms were seldom directed at local doctors, but rather 'the system'. Hospital experiences were frequently recounted as particularly alienating and unsympathetic, and for some individuals interviewed, the disclosure of bad news was recounted as being particularly insensitive and handled in an inappropriate manner.

Curers provided an alternative to unsuccessful medical consultations. At the most basic level, patients were able to describe and elaborate on symptoms at a pace, priority and manner that they themselves deemed important (thereby avoiding possible frustration of being unheard or misunderstood). Folk medicine also had the potential to question the authority and knowledge of the doctor and thereby act as a brake to practices that were regarded as unsound or that were not fully trusted.

In terms of efficacy, many people in both communities believed in the magical properties of the charm and thought that physiological changes can and did occur as a result of going for a cure. The possible outcomes of a cure/charm may be categorised in four ways. Firstly, they were regarded as having an actual physically beneficial effect. Secondly, they might be regarded as cathartic, producing a psychological effect, in that a sense of well-being was produced as a result of seeking a cure or knowing that one was about to go for a cure. Healers produced a 'feel good factor', effecting what Csordas and Kleinman have referred to as 'the talking cure' (Csordas and Kleinman 1996:15; cf. Koss-Chioino 2006). Even the knowledge that curers lived locally appeared to be of therapeutic value. Thirdly, cures might also be thought of as having a neutral effect, in that there was no real or perceived effect of any kind, though they did no harm. And fourthly, they could be thought of as having a negative effect, whereby delay in seeing a doctor because of the expectation of the effectiveness of a cure might actually worsen a serious health condition.

Among those interviewed in both towns, narratives overwhelmingly dwelt on the beneficial effects. Few addressed neutral effects and only one GP interviewed addressed the negative effects of the cure. Many of the healthcare professionals interviewed, while practicing scientific, formal, modern medicine, were familiar with folk medicine and both modes were factored into their practice in their professional and personal lives. While there was a pragmatic reliance on formal medicine for detailed information on specific conditions and some forms of potent medication, prescriptions and doctor's signatures for work or insurance claims, many in Ballymacross and Hunterstown regarded formal medicine as remote and often uninterested in their case.

On the face of it, much of the social science literature points to the emergence, dominance and monopoly of Western biomedicine and how this has successfully marginalised folk health systems. In the cases of Ballymacross and Hunterstown, this was not so. The lay and professional community in both towns studied show that, rather than being marginalised, folk healing practices were integral to health services in the locale. While they may not have had officially sanctioned legitimacy, they were not without authority. Scientific medicine and ethnomedicine may be underpinned by contrasting ideologies. This research suggests that these ideologies did not only coexist but were codependent on one another. Local people in Ballymacross and Hunterstown applied a pragmatic rationale to health needs and used folk and formal medicine in a complementary and interchangeable fashion. Both healthcare systems were utilised and managed by local people and health professionals alike. Catholic Ballymacross and Protestant Hunterstown illustrate a system of medical pluralism and pragmatic eclecticism where there was a tacit understanding of the principles of, and the value of, both formal and informal healing. As a result, healthcare in both towns was characterised by this.

Folk healing practices also had benefits beyond the individual and the medical. Belief in the cure/charm was symbolically central to both communities. This appeared more visible in Ballymacross, which illustrated a specifically Catholic flavour, and appeared to add to a sense of local identity. It also contributed to a sense of social solidarity. Belief in the cure, while not being specifically Christian, supported a religious (and culturally Catholic) ethos. In Hunterstown, folk healing was less important as a means of reifying culture (although curative practices did represent a reaffirmation of community), but its significance lay in it being a challenge and alternative to modern health practices deemed problematic and unsympathetic. In a general sense, the cure was also understood simultaneously as a gift (from the curer to the person, and from the community to the individual), and a transaction (in return, local people continued the tradition).

The cure/charm acted as a form of social support (and cognitive therapy) emphasizing ritual and culture, social bonds and neighbourliness. The belief was public, yet the acts were private. Belief in the cure was part of a social commitment and in this sense it was the mortar binding a distinct and fundamental value system, in these communities. This influenced social behaviour, social regulation and approval. Curing is required and sanctioned by the community. The healer cures because of the beliefs and practices traditionally understood in these communities and because people want and expect healers to cure them. In this sense the cure lies not with the curer but with the community at large. Some cures were recognised as more overtly religious, such as occasional trips to Lourdes for devout Ballymacross Catholics (and Protestants), or faith healing from a Pentecostal pastor in Hunterstown. But mostly, cures/charms were not bound by spirituality or religious affiliation. Cosmologically, cures were tied to ecological factors, to local culture and to the local economy. Cures/charms were to this extent extra-religious.

Cures and charms are not exotic belief systems, they are not even subterranean health systems; rather, they are alive and their mechanisms are understood not only in metaphor but also in action. This distinct form of folk healing has survived the Reformation and the Industrial Revolution and is resistant to various expressions of high modernity, including globalisation and cosmopolitanism.

Notes

1. The research on which this chapter is based was funded by the Department of Health and Social Services (Northern Ireland) and I would like to thank them for financing the initial research project into Health Inequalities in two Northern Ireland Communities. Northern Ireland makes up the largest proportion of one of four provinces in Ireland, and is known as Ulster. The names used for the two communities on which this chapter focuses – Ballymacross and Hunterstown – are pseudonyms, and by saying that these are 'predominantly' Catholic and Protestant communities respectively, I mean that these religious identifications apply to more than 80 per cent of the population in each case.
2. A full discussion of this can be found in Moore (1996).
3. Kleinman (1980) offers a discussion of how this operates as a health system.

4. Scottish and English settlers colonized the Northern province of Ulster during the early part of the seventeenth century.
5. The Orange Order is a pan-Protestant organisation that united Protestants from various social and denominational backgrounds in defence against the threat of an all-Ireland, Catholic-dominated Republic.
6. The annual Protestant demonstration/celebration of 12 July is an example of this.
7. The terms 'ritual' or 'magic' are not used by the curers themselves or their patients, 'but 'the use of the term "charm" has magical connotations for people who themselves do not possess a cure' (Buckley 1980: 22).
8. The physician David Rorie spent most of his life in rural Northeast Scotland and documented local, folk medical practices from the late 1800s to the 1930s. He well understood the difference between 'lofty learning' and local cultural practice and the central role folk healing and folk medicine played in community life.
9. See Hamilton (2001) for a good outline and excellent critical discussion of Durkheim's position.
10. In recent years public trust has become a major point of scrutiny for social theorists (see, e.g., Beck 1992).
11. Lawrence (1985) argues that in the Victorian and Edwardian eras this apparent unity was tenuous. Rather, the profession was variegated in its attitudes, goals and standards, and especially in its definition, evaluation and use of science.
12. The cultural gap between biomedical practitioners and patients is also discussed by Bakx (1991).

References

Anderson, B. 1983. *Imagined Communities: Reflections on the Origin and Spread of Nationalism*. London: Verso.

Bakx, K. 1991. 'The "Eclipse' of Folk Medicine in Western Society', *Sociology of Health and Illness* 13(1): 20–38.

Beck, U. 1992. *Risk Society: Towards a New Modernity*. London: Sage.

Lady Wilde nd: *Irish Cures, Mystic Charms and Superstition* Barry, S. 1990. New York: Stirling. Compiled from, Ancient legends, mystic charms, and superstitions of Ireland 1826-1896 nd, and Ancient cures, charms, and usages of Ireland nd. Both by Lady Wilde.

Buchan, D. (ed.) 1994. *Folk Traditions and Folk Medicine in Scotland: The Writings of David Rorie*. Edinburgh: Canongate Academic.

Buckley, T. 1980. 'Unofficial Healing in Ulster', in A. Gailey (ed.) *Ulster Folklife*. Newry: Ulster Folk and Transport Museum.

Bynum, W. F. and R. Porter 1993. Companion Encyclopedia of the History of Medicine, Vol 2, London and New York: Routledge.

Csordas, T.J. and A. Kleinman. 1996. 'The Therapeutic Process', in C.F. Sargent and T.M. Johnson (eds), *Medical Anthropology: Contemporary Theory and Method*. Westport, CT: Praeger.

DoH. 1992. 'The Health of The Nation: A Strategy for Health in England'. London: HMSO for the Department of Health.

DHSS. 1995. The Regional Strategy for Health and Social Well-being, 1997–2002. Belfast: Department of Health and Social Security, Northern Ireland.

Durkheim, E. 1915. *The Elementary Forms of Religious Life*. London: Allen and Unwin.

Fleetwood, J. 1983[1951]. *The History of Medicine in Ireland*. Dublin: Skelling Press.

Geertz, C. 1966. 'Religion as a Cultural System', in M. Banton (ed) *Anthropological Approaches to the Study of Religion*. London: Tavistock.

Giddens, A. (1990) *The Consequences of Modernity* Cambridge: Polity Press.

Graham, J. 1985. 'Folk Medicine and Intercultural Diversity among West Texas Mexican Americans', *Western Folklore* 44(3): 168–93.

Harris, R. 1972. *Prejudice and Tolerance in Ulster: A Study of Neighbours and 'Strangers' in a Border Community*. Manchester: Manchester University Press.

Hamilton, M. 2001. *The Sociology of Religion*. London: Routledge.

Helman, C. 2007. *Culture, Health and Illness*. London: Hodder Arnold.

Howe, L. 1990. *Being Unemployed in Northern Ireland: An Ethnographic Study*. Cambridge: Cambridge University Press.

Kleinman, A. (1980). Patients and healers in the context of culture: an exploration of the borderland between anthropology, medicine, and psychiatry. Berkeley: University of California Press.

———. 1993. 'Concepts and a Model for the Comparison of Medical Systems as Cultural Systems', in C. Currer and M. Stacey (eds), *Concepts of Health, Illness and Disease: A Comparative Perspective*. Oxford: Berg.

Koss-Chioino, J. 2006. 'Spiritual Transformation, Relation and Radical Empathy: Core Components of the Ritual Healing Process', *Transcultural Psychiatry* 43(4): 652–70.

Landy, D. 1974. 'Role Adaptation: Traditional Curers under the Impact of Western Medicine', *American Ethnologist* 1(1): 103–27.

Larsen, S. 1982 'The two sides of the house: identity and social organisation', 131-64 in P Cohen (ed.) Belonging: Identity and Social Organisation in British Rural Culture. Manchester: Manchester University Press.

Lawrence, C. 1985. 'Incommunicable Knowledge: Science, Technology and the Clinical Art in Britain', *Journal of Contemporary History* 20(4): 503–20.

Logan, P. 1981. *Irish Country Cures*. Belfast: Appletree Press.

Lundy, P. and M. McGovern. 2007. 'Catholic Habitus and Identity in Northern Ireland', in S. O'Sullivan (ed.) *Contemporary Ireland: A Sociological Map*. Dublin: UCD Press.

Macfarlane, A. (1998). 'Medical Pluralism In Ireland 1930s–1990s', unpublished Ph.D. thesis. Galway: National University Of Ireland.

Macfarlane, A. and P. Ginnety. 2001. 'Boiled Nettles in May: Studies of Plural Medicine in Northern and Southern Ireland', in M. Maclachlan (ed.) *Cultivating Health: Cultural Perspectives On Promoting Health*. Chichester: Wiley and Sons.

Moore, R. 2004. 'Lambegs and Bodhrans: Religion, Identity and Health in Northern Ireland', in D. Kelleher and G. Leavey (eds), *Identity and Health*. London: Routledge.

______. 2007. Protestants and Protestant Habitus in Northern Ireland', in S. O'Sullivan (ed.) *Contemporary Ireland: A Sociological Map*. Dublin: UCD Press.

Moore, R., S. Harrisson, C. Mason and J. Orr. 1996. The Use of an Ethnographic Approach to Assessment of Health Need in Northern Ireland', *Nursing Times Research* 1(4): 251–59.

______. 1997a. 'Inequalities in Health in Two Northern Ireland Communities and Assessment of Related Need', unpublished report for the Department of Health and Social Services in Northern Ireland. Belfast: Queen's University.

______. 1997b. 'Health Professionals' Perspectives on Service Delivery in Northern Ireland', unpublished report for the Department of Health and Social Services in Northern Ireland. Belfast: Queen's University.

Moore, R. and A. Sanders. 1996. 'The Limits of and Anthropology of Conflict?: Loyalist and Republican Paramilitary Organisations In Northern Ireland', in A. Wolfe and H. Yang (eds), *Anthropological Approaches to Conflict Resolution*. Athens: University of Georgia Press.

Murphy, A. and C Kelleher 1995 Contemporary heath practices in the Burren. *Irish Journal of Psychology*, 16, 38–51.

Murtagh, B. 1996. Community and Conflict in Rural Ulster: A Study of Belfast's Peace Lines. Centre for the Study of Conflict Publication, University of Ulster.

O'Reilly, D. and M. Stevenson. 1998. 'The Two Communities in Northern Ireland: Depression and Ill health', *Journal of Public Health Medicine* 20(2): 161–68.

Porter, R. 2000. *The Greatest Benefit to Mankind: A Medical History of Humanity*. London: Norton.

Robson, B., M. Bradford and I. Dees. 1994. *Relative Deprivation in Northern Ireland*. Manchester: Centre for Urban Policy Studies, Manchester University.

Roch, A. 1981. 'Folk Medicine and Faith Healing in Northern Ireland', unpublished Ph.D. thesis. Belfast: Department of Anthropology, Queen's University.

Stringer, P. 1990. 'Spatial and Social Variations in the Distribution of Health Indicators in Northern Ireland', unpublished report for the Department of Health and Social Services in Northern Ireland. Belfast: Policy Institute and Northern Ireland Research Laboratory, University of Ulster/Queen's University.

Chapter 6
Rescuing Folk Remedies: Ethnoknowledge and the Reinvention of Indigenous Herbal Medicine in Britain

Ayo Wahlberg

Obtain [a] 7lb toffee jar and pack the comfrey leaves as tight as you can in it. Then forget it for at least six months. The leaves will have become a ball of 'Goo' and I add stink to high heaven. Pour the liquid into a much smaller jar for immediate use as a cure for sprains and the like. Leave the old stuff in the large jar and top up with new leaves the following year. Now how true this next bit of info is I'm not sure. But the 'know-alls' reckon that the second growing of the plant –first leaves are from about March, the second from around August – these are the true healing ones. To me they are both the same, and stink just as badly.

–H.G.

Neem is very good, because I'm diabetic, it helps me to control my diabetes. My friend has managed to get me some neem leaves from India, and I have been using it to control my diabetes. I mix it with my tea and I drink it, it keeps the sugar level down. I remember when I was little, I had chicken pox, and my mother kept me indoors for 3 days and then she boiled some neem leaves in water. And she washed me with it and I was fine.

–S.M.

If there is one thing that is agreed upon in the otherwise highly contested field of herbal medicine, it is that peoples and cultures all over the world have been using plants to treat their ailments for a very long time – the proverbial roots of medicine. This has certainly been the case in the British Isles and indeed there is a long history of organised herbal medicine practice which survives to this day.[1] Ever since the founding of the National Association of Medical Herbalists in 1864 (later the National Institution of Medical Herbalists, NIMH), around the same time that the General Medical Council was established in the United Kingdom following the 1858 Medical Act, learned herbal practitioners have had their schools, codes of practice and representative organisations. Yet, despite this legacy of formalisation, it is only as recently as 2001 that statutory recognition became a realistic option for herbal practitioners. In the intervening century and a half, organised herbal practice suffered numerous defeats as well as more or less concerted actions to wipe it out by lawmakers and biomedical professional organisations (Brown 1985; Saks 1992; Griggs 1997).

There has, however, always been another side to herbal medicine in the British Isles, namely folk remedies and family healing. These are all those home recipes for aches, pains, rashes and 'nerves' which have been prepared in British kitchens for centuries, often passed down orally from mother (mostly) or father to daughter or son and some times recorded in a rich archive of herbals, some of which became bestsellers in their time with others remaining within family circles in the form of 'kitchen books' (Hatfield 2005). It is also these very same remedies that over time have been variously accorded the discourteous labels of 'old wives' tales', 'superstitions' or 'folk beliefs'. Yet in the last century or two, massive transformations in British society resulting from processes of industrialisation and urbanisation, and more recently globalisation, are feared to have put knowledge of indigenous folk remedies at grave risk of extinction. To begin with, a good part of herbal medicine has itself come to be modernised and industrialised to such an extent that a new generation of urban or 'black-bottle herbalists'[2] are seen by some to be at risk of losing touch with the land. Moreover, oral traditions of handing down family remedies are seen to be rapidly dying out as a growing proportion of British people come to live in busy urban settings where quick-fix, over-the-counter pharmaceuticals are readily available for day-to-day aches and blues. And finally, following decades of transatlantic and continental influence, the ongoing consolidation of a multiethnic Britain has meant that herbal medicine is no longer solely practiced in its Western form. As a consequence, medicinal plants are increasingly being imported, particularly in urban centres, to stock not just the practices of traditional Chinese, Ayurvedic or Tibetan medicine, but also of Western practitioners of herbal medicine who have integrated imported Asian and Latin American species into their repertoire of healing plants. Amidst such a pluralisation of herbal practice in Britain, British herbal medicine has had in a sense to reinvent itself as 'Western herbal medicine'.[3]

In this chapter, I will examine how one might account for the much-celebrated late-twentieth-century revival of herbal medicine in the U.K. According to the NIMH, 'enthusiasm for this ancient form of medicine has never been greater than it is today' (NIMH 2007), a revival that is often traced back to the 1968 Medicines Act. In sociological studies of complementary and alternative medicine (CAM) it has been commonly suggested that it is in the failures of biomedicine that we can find the origins of the interest in and take-up of not only herbal medicine but also many other forms of complementary, alternative or folk medicine, such as acupuncture, homeopathy, osteopathy and aromatherapy. In these accounts, the reductionism, dehumanisation, toxins and alienation associated with an impersonal and bureaucratised health service reliant on biomedicine are seen as symptomatic of a broader range of side effects attributed to 'modern life' emerging from processes of modernisation, urbanisation, industrialisation and globalisation (see Coward 1989; Sharma 1992; O'Connor 1995; Cant and Sharma 1996). It is as antidotes to the life-enfeebling and soul-battering side effects of modernity that forms of complementary and folk medicine have in recent decades been promoted. As such, the revival of herbal medicine in the British Isles taps into a much broader critique of modern society which spans concerns about the negative impact of increasing environmental degradation and pollution as well as processes of clinical, social and cultural iatrogenesis that are seen to have transformed individuals 'into unfeeling spectators of their own decaying selves' (Illich 1976: 35; see also Szersynski 2005).

Indeed, some have argued that herbal medicine may well be another victim of this if ongoing efforts to professionalise and modernise it are not put on hold. Herbalist Peter Jackson-Main has argued that '[b]y defining herbal medicine as a graduate entry profession, there is a danger that the emphasis on academic learning may eclipse traditional values and practices' (Jackson-Main 2005: 97), while Jagtenberg and Evans have suggested that '[i]n a rapidly changing field, it is globalization that comes in the guise of science, technology, and progress that is more likely to destabilise the traditions of Western herbal medicine' (Jagtenberg and Evans 2003: 325).

Somewhat in contrast, what I will be arguing in this chapter is that what might be thought of as the disciplining and normalisation of herbal medicine have been integral to its revival in the U.K. The point I will be making is that processes of industrialisation, professionalisation and modernisation should not be seen as somehow antithetical to an 'authentic' herbal medicine, but instead be seen as elements of its ongoing recasting and rectification (cf. Canguilhem 1988; Bachelard 2001). This is not say that there is no such thing as 'good' herbal medicine as compared to 'bad' herbal medicine; rather, it is to say that what is considered 'good' and 'bad' in any kind of medicine is a problem which is historically locatable and dependent on social practices and procedures for validating, assuring and safeguarding, practices which in turn are always subject to contestation and rectification.

In what follows, I will show how herbal medicine came to be actively reinvented in the U.K. from about the mid twentieth century onwards. The analysis is based primarily on documents from herbal medicine practitioner associations, official government bodies, individual herbal practitioners and ethnobotanists, as well as from various interdisciplinary initiatives such as the Remembered Remedies and Plant Cultures projects. There are three parts to the chapter: the first concerns longstanding attempts to unify what has been described as a fragmented group of herbal medicine practitioner associations; the second concerns the twentieth-century transformation of herbals into pharmacopoeias and the resulting emergence of 'herbal medicinal products' as a new legal category; and the final part concerns urgent efforts to record oral herbal traditions before they die out amidst increasing urbanisation and globalisation. What will be a consistent theme throughout this chapter is that of ambivalence towards what 'modern life' in the U.K. has to offer herbal medicine and vice versa. It should be noted that it will not be a part of this chapter's remit to evaluate whether herbal medicine in the U.K. is better or worse off today compared to any other point in history. What I will instead be empirically accounting for are some of the conditions of possibility that have made space for herbal medicine's recent 'renaissance in the modern world' (Mills 1993: 17).

Fragmentation and the Disciplining of Herbal Practice

As already noted, the organisation of herbal medicine practitioners into associations, which look after the interests and training of its members in Britain, goes back at least to 1864 when the National Association of Medical Herbalists (now NIMH) was formed. And ever since its Memorandum of Association came into force in 1895, they have distinguished between qualified and unqualified herbalists, actively sought 'to train Medical Herbalists', worked 'to repress malpractices', as well as investigated cases of 'unprofessional conduct' through a General Council of Safe Medicine (NIMH 1979; Brown 1985). In lobbying for a Medical Herbalists Bill in the early part of the twentieth century, the Association argued that 'it is our desire to compel a standard of Education and Registration so that the public shall be enabled to differentiate between Bona Fide [sic] Herbalists and those who trade on the name' (cited in Griggs 1997: 262).[4] Yet this distinction did not gain any kind of official sanctioning during the first half of the twentieth century and was firmly opposed by the medical establishment (Wahlberg 2007b). The proposed Medical Herbalists Bill (which would have given herbal practitioners statutory recognition as a medical profession on a par with biomedical doctors) was denied by the British Ministry of Health in 1923, among others, on the grounds that it is 'doubtful whether a trained herbalist is any less dangerous than an untrained one' (chief medical officer, cited in Larkin 1992: 117). In an increasingly hostile environment, the herbal practitioners from the National Association of Medical Herbalists also struggled to finance a herbal medicine school that could ensure consistent training standards for its members. Then, in 1941, a new Pharmacy and Medicines Act revoked the right of herbalists in the U.K. to supply herbal medicines directly to patients on the grounds of protecting the public, in effect making it illegal for herbal practitioners to practice. Indeed, Griggs has argued that what British herbalists faced between the end of the nineteenth and middle of the twentieth century was nothing short of 'continuous ... harassment, vexation and attempted legal suppression by the medical establishment' (Griggs 1997: 234).[5] The situation had become so dire by the late 1960s that, as Griggs notes, there were only a handful of 'formally' apprentice-trained medical herbalists left.

All this would change, however, in 1968 when, following intense lobbying, medical herbalists secured the so-called 'Section 12 exemptions' in a new Medicines Act. This relieved herbal remedies provided through one-to-one consultations with herbalists, and 'traditionally prepared' over-the-counter herbal medicines, of the expensive safety and quality requirements that other medicinal products had to adhere to. Quite soon hereafter, sales of herbal medicines, the number of schools providing training in herbalism, and consultations with herbalists, all grew in tandem with an otherwise growing crisis of modern medicine (Griggs 1997; Saks 2003; O'Sullivan 2005). By the end of the twentieth century, herbal medicine was considered to be among the 'big five' of complementary and alternative medicines in terms of prevalence of use and practice, alongside osteopathy, chiropractic, homeopathy and acupuncture (House of Lords 2000). It is precisely this increased use of herbal medicine, coupled with traditions of self-regulation dating back to the formation of the NIMH, as well as herbal safety issues arising from the Section 12 exemptions, that would make it a priority candidate (following on from the statutory recognition of osteopathy and chiropractic in 1993 and 1994 respectively) for recent regulatory efforts to protect the public from its 'dangerous and incompetent' practice at the turn of the millennium (see House of Lords 2000; Wahlberg 2007b).

The NIMH, by far the largest of herbal practitioner organisations today with over 500 members (DoH et al. 2003: 12), has in many ways pre-empted the debates which since the 1980s have increasingly placed practitioner competency and qualifications at the heart of the 'CAM question' (see BMA 1986, 1993; House of Lords 2000). Already in 1991, the NIMH introduced a binding Code of Ethics, Code of Practice and Disciplinary Procedures, which was followed up by the formation of an NIMH Accreditation Board in 1994 to assess standards in the training of medical herbalists. And, the title of 'medical herbalist' has itself always served to distinguish trained practitioners from lay practitioners.

Training to become a medical herbalist by an NIMH-accredited institution in the U.K. today includes courses in the theories and practices of both herbal and biomedicine, including anatomy, physiology and pathology, not least because:

> If we want to continue to enjoy our right in this country for trained Medical Herbalists to have the right of primary diagnosis (a licence which is unique in Europe and perhaps even in the 'developed' world), we have to acquire a high level of orthodox clinical skills. To this end, the first two years of the course contain, alongside Herbal Science, a fair degree of Anatomy, Physiology and Pathology. (Scottish School of Herbal Medicine 2006)

Yet the NIMH has not been alone in endeavours to organise and train herbal practitioners. The last century and more has seen the formation (and in some cases demise) of a Society of United Medical Herbalists of Great Britain (1877), a Society of Herbalists (1927), a Botano-Therapuetic Institute (1931), an International Register of Consultant Herbalists (1960), a British Herbal Medicine Association (1964), a College of Practitioners of Phytotherapy (1982),[6] and an Association of Master Herbalists (1996). Common to these many different organisations has been the fact that most of their members have been practitioners of a tradition of herbal medicine indigenous to Britain (albeit with abundant transatlantic and continental influences and interactions) whose father figures include Gerard, Culpeper and Coffin. Yet the members of these organisations have not necessarily always seen eye to eye, with some suggesting that a rationalised phytomedicine or 'black-bottle' herbal medicine is the best way forward and others resisting the growing industrialisation and modernisation of the cultivation and production of herbal remedies (see Brown 1985; Griggs 1997; Jagtenberg and Evans 2003).

More recently, an additional component of new medical pluralism has manifested itself in the U.K., with the consolidation of various herbal medical practices rooted in the cultural traditions of immigrant ethnic communities, such as Ayurveda, traditional Chinese and traditional Tibetan medicine. Consequently, during the past two decades, a Register of Chinese Herbal Medicine (1987), a College of Tibetan Medicine (1993), an Association of Traditional Chinese Medicine (1994), an Ayurvedic Medical Association (1996), a British Ayurvedic Medical Council (1999), a British Society of Chinese Medicine (2001), and even a Unified Register of Herbal Practitioners(1997)[7] have also been formed. Indeed, it was as these different organisations were establishing themselves throughout the late 1980s and 1990s that the term 'Western herbal medicine' was coined to cover a tradition of herbal medicine particular to North America, Great Britain and Australia.

In 2001, a Herbal Medicine Regulatory Working Group was formed as a joint initiative of the Department of Health, the Prince of Wales's Foundation for Integrated Health (PWFIH) and the European Herbal Practitioners Association (EHPA). One of its key tasks was to address this plurality and fragmentation. The Working Group, which further includes representation from no fewer than eleven herbal medicine organisations representing some 1,500 practitioners, was given a mandate to come up with proposals for the statutory regulation of the herbal medicine profession as a whole. In 2003, the group published a range of recommendations for how a self-regulated council of some form could be given the legal right to determine minimum levels of competence for those wishing to be registered as 'medical herbalists' (with due specifications for Western, Chinese and Ayurvedic forms of it), standards of ethical and responsible practice of herbal medicine, as well as disciplinary mechanisms for excluding and/or penalising 'unacceptable professional conduct' by registered herbalists (DoH et al. 2003: 17–21).

Thus, an important part of the herbal-medicine revival in the UK has been a series of efforts to finally officially sanction what an albeit fragmented group of herbal practitioners, led by the NIMH, had been lobbying for since the nineteenth century: a state-sanctioned mechanism to enable the public 'to differentiate between Bona Fide [sic] Herbalists and those who trade on the name'. What is more, the fragmentation that has characterised herbal medicine practice for centuries in the U.K. would take on a new twist in the globalising 1990s as a whole range of 'non-Western' therapies became established features of especially urban centres. At the time of writing (summer 2009), herbal medicine was in line to become only the third non-biomedical therapy (following osteopathy and chiropractic) to become statutorily recognised in the U.K.

From Herbals to Pharmacopoeias

It is an oft-cited wisdom that if a remedy is still around after centuries of documented use, then there must be something to it. It is common in contemporary literature about herbal medicine to see references to its use by 'ancient civilisations' some '3,000 years ago' (Chevallier 1999: 81; cf. Mills 1993: 5). Yet such persistent invocation of longstanding use has also led regulators at the Department of Health to argue that 'the medical herbalist is at fault for clinging to outworn historical authority and for not assessing his drugs in terms of today's knowledge' (cited in BMA 1986: 110). This tension between historical authority (continuity with an ancient past) and scientific authority (the need to re-evaluate herbal medicine in light of present knowledge) was recently captured in the European Council Directive on traditional herbal medicinal products which argued that a long tradition of use 'makes it possible to reduce the need for clinical trials, in so far as the efficacy of the [herbal] medicinal product is *plausible* on the basis of long-standing use and experience' while also insisting that 'even a long tradition does not exclude the possibility that there may be concerns with regard to the product's safety ... [and] quality' (European Parliament 2004: 5, emphasis added). It is a tension that has also characterised the revival of herbal medicine in the U.K.

As is the case in many other parts of the world, the British Isles are home to a rich archive of books describing plants and their medicinal properties, known as 'herbals'. They can be found scattered throughout the past centuries of publishing history, from John Gerard's *Herball or General Historie of Plantes* (1597), Nicholas Culpeper's *The English Physitian* (1652), Elizabeth Blackwell's *A Curious Herbal* (1739), William Withering's *A Botanical Arrangement of all the Vegetables Naturally Growing in Great Britain* (1776),

Robert John Thornton's *A Family Herbal* (1814), to Albert Isaiah Coffin's *A Botanic Guide to Health and the Natural Pathology of Disease* (1852). The result of meticulous study by their authors, these oft-reprinted books and many other similar herbals have been instrumental in the subsequent botanical identification, classification and description of medicinally used British plant species. Yet, it was these very books that would end up banished to the fringes of medicine by the end of the nineteenth century, rejected by a growing medical profession as nothing more than collections of old wives' tales that still relied on the doctrine of signatures or astrology for explanations of efficacy. And although the synthetic drugs of modern medicine were ironically enough often developed through the isolation and chemical transformation of single active compounds found in plants, medical doctors were quick to contrast their 'purified' medicines with the 'messy' or 'impure' remedies of herbalists as part of their marginalising strategies.

At any rate, it was precisely to counter such charges that herbalists set about publishing a series of updated reference books in the early part of the twentieth century. In 1905 the National Association of Medical Herbalists published the first *National Botanic Pharmacopoeia*. Fifteen years later, Mathew Robinson published *The New Family Herbal* (1920), in which he claimed that any notion of 'the government of Herbs by the sun, moon and planets, has been exploded by modern science; and is now regarded by persons of ordinary capacity to be absurd in the extreme' (cited in Brown 1985: 81). A few years later, Maud Grieve and Hilda Leyel published what they called *A Modern Herbal*, arguing that,

> All serious Herbalists have long realized that a new Herbal is badly needed – a herbal which must include the traditional lore and properties of plants, *and* the modern use of properly standardized extracts and tinctures which were unknown in the days of Gerard and Parkinson, and even in the days of Culpeper, and which have been made possible by the development of modern chemistry. (Grieve and Leyel 1931: 3, emphasis added)

These updated reference books covering more than 800 herbs – listed according to botanical name, botanical family, synonyms, parts used, botanical description, constituents, indications, medicinal action, medicinal uses, preparation and dosage – marked important steps in the transformation of the long-standing 'herbal' into a monograph-based pharmacopoeia of herbs and herbal remedies. It was a transformation that relied on a comprehensive mapping-out exercise of botanical enlightenment, designed to put order into the rich yet sometimes chaotic, unsystematic, unscientific and even unwritten records of medicinal herbs that have been used for centuries.

It would not, however, be until 1965 that efforts to prepare the current *British Herbal Pharmacopoeia* began. As Griggs (1997: 281–85) has shown, during the drafting of the 1968 Medicines Act, the British Herbal Medicine Association (BHMA) – an interest group of herbalists, manufacturers and retailers formed in 1964 – had been informed that 'a herb for which a monograph appeared in any standard reference book and was not poisonous' might be exempted from the kind of evidence requirements for safety and efficacy that were a precondition for pharmaceutical medicines seeking market authorisation. What is more, while the 1968 Medicines Act did end up exempting from licensing those non-industrially produced herbal remedies sold without any written recommendations as to their use, manufacturers of herbal remedies were not exempt from an obligation to ensure quality and were thus in urgent need of a scientific reference book to which they could refer.

In response, the BHMA quickly put together a Scientific Committee in 1965 made up of pharmacologists, botanists, pharmacists and physicians, who were set the task of bringing order to the rich, yet dispersed and sometimes outdated, information that was available from the various herbals, as well as other sources of literature on the safety, efficacy and also quality of various medicinal plants. Their work comprised of enlightening forays into a variety of herbals, recorded case studies and journal articles, in order to chase up bibliographic leads and systematically map out individual medicinal plants according to available information on their botanical description, vernacular names, medicinal uses, history, chemistry, indications, side effects and recommended dosages.

The fruits of the BHMA Scientific Committee's labours came in the form of the first *British Herbal Pharmacopoeia*, which was published in stages starting with 115 herbal monographs in 1976 followed by a further 83 in 1979 and 34 in 1981 (Griggs 1997: 282–83). The *British Herbal Pharmacopoeia* was the first of its kind in the West, but has since been followed up in Germany, where 380 monographs were published by Commission E in the period 1983 to 1995;[8] in the U.S.A., where the development of an *American Herbal Pharmacopoeia* was initiated in 1994; at the European level, where the European Scientific Cooperative on Phytotherapy published 60 monographs in the period 1997 to 1999; and more recently at the international level with the World Health Organization publication of three volumes of monographs on selected medicinal plants, published since 1999.

The point to be made is that whereas herbals and treatises have undoubtedly played a key role in the identification and classification of medicinally useful herbs, the aim of monograph-based pharmacopoeias has been much more one of assurance and safeguarding. That is to say, while herbals and their authors continue to be celebrated for the important contributions they have made, these herbals certainly do not constitute authoritative references on issues of safety, quality and efficacy as far as regulatory authorities are concerned. As the British Pharmacopoeia Commission recently argued, a 'monograph, taken as a whole, should provide a reliable basis for making an independent judgement as to the quality of the substance in the interests of the protection of the public' (BPC 2004). Hence, the ordering and updating of information on medicinal plants and herbal remedies – as witnessed in the mapping-out efforts of medical herbalists and pharmacologists in the U.K. and indeed throughout the world – and the conversion or updating of herbals and treatises into monograph-based pharmacopoeias, has been a crucial part of the ongoing revival of herbal medicine.

At the same time, further to consolidating a documented reference base, the emergence of herbal pharmacopoeias has also facilitated twentieth-century efforts to standardise and modernise herbal remedies. While leaflets and packaging labels in, for example, Holland and Barrett outlets often present herbal medicinal products as '100% natural!', 'organic', 'conventionally grown' or 'wild crafted', a lot has happened since the days of John Gerard, Nicholas Culpeper and Albert Coffin. Over the past century or so, medicinal plant cultivation and processing has been transformed into a highly technologised, multi-million-dollar industry (Richter 2003). Inspired by the pioneering work of German natural-product chemists and companies in the 1920s and 1930s,[9] the industrialisation of medicinal plants into what have come to be known as 'phytomedicines' has developed into a global activity with supply chains spanning all the world's continents. Indeed, the late-twentieth-century boom in herbal medicine, often cited as evidence of the growing popularity of alternative and traditional medicines, refers in large part to rapid rises in the sales figures for phytomedicines throughout the 1980s and 1990s (see Gaedcke and Steinhoff 2002; Richter 2003). As a result, as any herbalist will point out today, it is important to distinguish on the one hand between mass-produced phytomedicines, which are often standardised against a certain single active ingredient (such as hypericin or hyperforin, found in St John's wort) on the one hand, and the dried, comminuted or crushed starting materials (leaves, buds, flowers, stems, bark, and so forth) from which extracts and tinctures are prepared by medical herbalists in consultations (or by herbal remedy producers such as Neal's Yard Remedies) on the other. Where quality was in the past (and to some extent continues to be by some medical herbalists) controlled by an individual herbalist who strolled the countryside, smelling and feeling the texture of medicinal plants before plucking them; today, quality is often controlled in high-tech laboratories against plant-constituent profiles known as liquid chromatographic 'fingerprints' (see Jagtenberg and Evans 2003; Wahlberg 2008b).

Nevertheless, whether in the form of its original starting material (fresh, dried or comminuted leaves, stems, flower buds or bark) or as industrially produced capsules, tonics or tablets, herbal medicines that are sold for health-related purposes and/or make health-related curative claims have increasingly become subject to safety and standardisation requirements as a means to assure users and to protect them from the potential dangers that are both inherent to the 'natural' herbs but also augmented by industrial production practices in the form of contamination and adulteration risks. If we look at the past few decades worth of measures to regulate the production and sale of herbal medicinal products in the U.K., it is clear that safety and quality concerns have been at the fore, much more so than the purported (lack of) efficacy of these products. In the wake of increasing sales of herbal medicine products, and in contrast to claims of a gentler, kinder and more natural herbal medicine, regulatory authorities are increasingly advising consumers, firstly, that 'natural does not necessarily mean safe' and, secondly, that in some cases these medicines are turning out to be 'not so natural after all'. A report from the UK Herbal Medicine Regulatory Working Group outlines the reasons why:

> For a long time … medicines law … left herbal medicine essentially unregulated in terms of quality and safety … But in recent years, along with a rapid expansion of the herbal sector, questions have arisen about the quality and safety of some herbal products. These questions have been variously associated with (a) adverse effects resulting from the inherent toxicity of certain herbal ingredients (natural does not always mean safe); (b) misidentification or substitution of one plant species for another, in some cases leading to the substitution of a safe with a toxic species; (c) adulteration of herbal medicines with prescription-only drugs or heavy metals; (d) microbial or fungal contamination of herbal remedies; (e) discovery of possible herb–drug interactions which may interfere with or confuse the results of treatment; (f) insufficient information provided to the consumer concerning the safe use of a herbal medicine. (DoH et al. 2004: 142)

And so, in the ways outlined here, the industrialisation of herbal medicine has certainly played an important role in the late-twentieth-century revival of herbal medicine, quite tangibly so as sales figures of herbal medicinal products are often used to verify the revival. At the same time, for many practising herbalists, this drift towards what is seen as 'rational phytotherapy' is something to be worried about. In many ways this tension is not resolvable, for how can an urban herbalist ensure quality when relying on medicinal plant products which may come from any corner of the world rather than on self-procured plants from the wild? Ready-made tinctures, capsules or tablets are no longer 'raw materials' but rather are 'herbal medicinal products' and as with any other mass-produced product, quality control is key. Herbal pharmacopoeias increasingly provide the technical details that can allow for a laboratory-based form of quality control and in the process they often identify particular active ingredients found in a plant as important markers of quality, even if herbalists insist that whole-plant extracts rather than single active ingredients are the key to ensuring safety and efficacy. As a result, the rationalisation and scientisation of herbal medicine is seen as necessary for a modern, urbanised U.K. by some and lamented by others who are concerned about a 'hollowing out' or 'reduction' of an 'authentic' and/or 'ancient' form of herbal medicine that is based on whole-plant extracts.

Documenting Wisdom: The Rise of Ethno-knowledge

As already noted, the formalised and rationalised practice and production of herbal medicine in Britain has only ever been one part of the story when it comes to herbal remedies and healing. Indeed, for much of the past two centuries it has arguably been the least important part, since rural populations in particular during the nineteenth and early twentieth centuries were often mostly self-reliant when it came to their daily medical needs (Hatfield 2005). Plants have long been the most important component of what Hatfield calls 'domestic medicine', which she describes as a 'do-it-yourself collection of first aid [for] mostly ordinary, often illiterate, country people' (ibid.: 9–10). While important components of the herbal-medicine revival have been the increasing formalisation and rationalisation of its practice and production, as we saw above, the majority of people who have used plants as medicine in the U.K. have not sought out trained herbalists for consultations; instead, they have relied on family remedies which were often passed down orally over the generations or perhaps recorded in ad hoc kitchen books which remained within families (Griggs 1997; Hatfield 2005). Even in contemporary urbanised Britain, it is striking to note that while some 7 per cent of people claim in recent surveys to have used herbal medicine in the past twelve months, only about 1 per cent say they have visited a herbalist for a consultation (House of Lords 2000: §1.17; O'Sullivan 2005: 184).

Still, it remains important to distinguish between an approach to herbal medicine where individuals get their remedies either through herbal consultations or more likely over the counter from high street outlets on the one hand, and an (albeit 'dying') domestic medicine on the other. On the urban front, it is interesting to note that the medical herbalist is highlighted as an expert who can assist otherwise unknowing consumers. For example, in an interview in 2002, the then president of the NIMH, Trudy Norris, cautioned that:

> What we are concerned about is that lots of people self-prescribe in an inappropriate way ... We are not against commercial herbal remedies bought for self-medication, but urge people to find out as much as possible before self-prescribing. In the market place matters of health and illness can create vulnerability. The practitioner's main focus is the actual health

needs of the patients over and above any consideration of profit. This cannot always be said of the entire supplement market. (BBC 2002)

Since then, an annual Herbal Medicine Awareness Week has been organised, a Herbal Health Advice Line has been opened to allow members of the public to get in touch with a local medical herbalist for expert advice, local walks with qualified herbalists to learn about the properties of medicinal plants growing in the U.K. and a revised edition of the booklet *Making Sense of Herbal Remedies* has been published advising consumers to choose their products carefully and to always seek advice from a qualified medical herbalist when in doubt (NIMH 2004; Norris 2004).

When it comes to domestic medicine, a much more profound transformation took place in the twentieth century, the effects of which can still be witnessed today. What Hatfield refers to as 'domestic medicine' would be called 'folk medicine' by many. But her choice of terminology is not accidental: 'the very word "folk" has come to have a patronising ring to it, and too often accounts of folk medicine concentrate on the bizarre and the fanciful. This has built up a picture of folk medicine as a collection of odd anachronistic rituals, practiced by the ignorant and superstitious' (Hatfield 2005: 5). For Hatfield, nothing could be further from the reality of rural Britain, as she has worked to systematically document how domestic medicine in fact 'represents the essence of plant wisdom of many centuries, and it is our loss if we dismiss this wisdom too lightly' (ibid.)

It is only in very recent years, through the efforts of ethnobotanists such as Gabrielle Hatfield and David Allen, as well as through multi-disciplinary initiatives such as Remembered Remedies and Plant Cultures, that 'folk' or 'domestic medicine' has come to be approached as a national treasure, as something with a value for the nation and therefore as something worth saving before it is lost to an increasingly urbanised, industrialised and globalised world. In 1999, a number of researchers from the Royal Botanical Gardens at Kew, the NIMH, the Herb Society, the Chelsea Physic Garden and Neal's Yard Remedies joined forces to form a research group called Ethnomedica. A few years later this group launched an urgent new programme which they called 'Remembered Remedies: Researching the Herbal Traditions of Britain'. Their rationale for doing so was clear:

> 150 years ago Britain was still mainly a rural society. Lives and activities were defined by the seasons and everyone knew the names and uses of several common wayside plants. Within two generations of the industrial revolution most of the population had moved into cities. As people developed an urban lifestyle they lost contact with the land and their practical herbal traditions. Not just forgotten but no longer accessible – where was the nearest dandelion, dock, healing tree or stream for watercress? … The loss of local knowledge – be it about plants or anything else – is one of the side effects of globalisation and rapidly changing societies. While this issue is recognised in the tropics, and is receiving a lot of attention from those concerned with development and the conservation of cultural and biological diversity, it is not the case here at home. The U.K. has long been industrialised and ranks among the most developed of regions. Yet studies have shown that fragments of knowledge passed down through a long oral tradition still exist among older people. Its value increases the more it is lost as time passes [sic]. (Ethnomedica 1999)

How then has it been possible for what, for many decades, were considered the old wives' tales, superstitions or folk beliefs of ignorant rural people to be transformed into a valued national resource worth documenting for posterity? To answer this question it is necessary to recount two crucial events within the discipline of anthropology in the twentieth century for reasons which will become clear. The first concerns an epistemological break with nineteenth-century evolutionary anthropology (see Wahlberg 2008a), and the second concerns the emergence of new methodologies with which to challenge evolutionary anthropology.

What is sometimes referred to as Victorian anthropology was informed and organised by an evolutionary logic. According to Spencer, Lubbock, Morgan and others, the world's peoples could be classified and ranked according to their collective states of maturity – as either civilised, barbarians or savages. The child-like simplicity and ignorance of 'savages', it was argued, was demonstrated by their rudimentary tools, monosyllabic languages and animistic religions (Wahlberg 2007a). Accordingly, what was described as 'primitive medicine' was seen as nothing more than superstitious ritual with little 'true' health benefits resulting for the 'savages' themselves. By the turn of the twentieth century, however, this logic came to be disputed by a new kind of anthropology which was based on cultural immersion and ethnography. Rivers, Malinowski, Boas and many others would reject the hypothesis that 'savages' were immature and simple, arguing instead, based on their in-depth field observations, that their practices and rituals were highly rational and informed by as complex a reasoning as that which could be found in the West. What was different was the world-views or life-worlds of people living in different cultures across the globe. As argued by Rivers: 'the practices of these peoples in relation to disease are not a medley of disconnected and meaningless customs, but are inspired by definite ideas concerning the causation of disease' (Rivers 1924: 52). Similarly, Erwin Ackerknecht wrote that 'primitive medicine is not a queer collection of errors and superstitions, but a number of living units in living cultural patterns, quite able to function through the centuries in spite of their fundamental differences from our own pattern' (Ackerknecht 1971: 120).

What these and other twentieth-century anthropologists needed then were new methodologies for accessing the life-worlds, ideas and cultural patterns of the people they studied. As a result, throughout the twentieth century, ethnographic methodologies of participant observation, in depth interviewing and overall immersion were developed and refined as a means of accessing the world-views of those peoples whose history was not documented in any archive. In Malinowski's famous phrase, the goal was 'to grasp the native's point of view, his relation to life, to realize his vision of his world' (Malinowski 1922: 25). At the same time, and in tandem with these developments in anthropology, the twentieth century also saw the rise of a whole range of new ethno-disciplines, from ethnobotany to ethnopharmacology and ethnoecology. What makes them 'ethno' sciences is their common focus on culturally transmitted traditional knowledge not only as a matter of cultural heritage, but also as an important ally in the search for ecologically, industrially and/or medically relevant plants or minerals. Their task is to document, through interviews, oral histories and participant observation, how certain groups or cultures use the flora and fauna around them for medical and other purposes.

Now, these two anthropological events –the disputing of evolutionary anthropology and the establishment of modern socio-cultural anthropology based on ethnographic fieldwork– have certainly had an effect in the British context when it comes to herbal medicine. To begin with, as Hatfield suggests, it is not only the 'savages' of faraway lands that have been considered 'simple' and 'ignorant' through the past centuries. Rural people in so-called 'civilised' countries have often been described in similar terms when contrasted to the 'educated', 'civilised' elite of the urban centres. It is these 'country people' who were seen as clinging on to outmoded, superstitious or backward healing remedies. So much so that, 'in our present century, elderly people with knowledge [of domestic medicine] usually have not passed it on to the next generation, for fear of being laughed at, or simply because they feel such information is not of interest to anyone' (Hatfield 2005: 12).

For projects like Remembered Remedies, it is exactly this information that is of great value and interest. In the three-year period 2003–2006, over one thousand records of medicinal plant use were gleaned from oral histories and survey cards that had been distributed widely by groups of researchers as well as by Kew Gardens. The Ethnomedica research group has trained over forty volunteer collectors through specialised training courses: 'The art of taking and recording an oral history is a specialized skill. It is more than listening, it is the task of hearing everything and collecting the details without prejudice or the need for them to make immediate sense; encouraging memories and reminiscences without leading' (Ethnomedica 1999). The information collected so far has been collated and organised, allowing researchers to produce a list of the top twenty most-mentioned plants (see Table 6.1). These included feverfew, dock, comfrey, onion, sage and nettle. Scientists at Kew have also been able to use the information gathered as a means of screening potential plant candidates for further phytochemical research into therapeutically active compounds. For example, Professor Monique Simmonds of Kew explains that 'sage is a herb that has been connected with wisdom down the ages, and now for the first time we can see whether it really helps with cognitive ability, or memory' (cited in Revill 2005).

Another project, Plant Cultures, is similarly using interviews and oral histories to document the uses and meanings of South Asian plants because 'Asian food, medicine, religion, music and film have all had a big impact on Britain's cultural landscape [and] British Asian communities form over 4% of the population of England and Wales, and over 25% of the population of cities such as Leicester' (Plant Cultures 2007). The project has listed twenty-five of the most popular plants such as chilli pepper, coconut, curry leaf and neem

Table 6.1: Top Twenty Plants Recorded by Ethnomedica, 2003–2008. Source: www.kew.org/ethnomedica/

Plant	Main use
Rumex – dock (377 records)	Stinging nettle
Allium cepa – onion (187 records)	Antibacterial
Urtica dioica – nettle (147 records)	Tonic; Rheumatism
Symphytum officinale – comfrey (126 records)	Bruising; bones
Sambucus nigra – elder (123 records)	Coughs and colds
Taraxacum officinale – dandelion (116 records)	Warts
Tanacetum parthenium – Feverfew (78 records)	Migraine
Brassica oleracea – cabbage (71 records)	Mastitis
Chamaemelum nobile (65 records)	Sleep
Citrus limon – lemon (59 records)	Coughs and colds
Allium sativum – garlic (57 records)	Antibacterial
Lavandula x *intermedia* – lavender (57 records)	Insommnia
Salvia officinalis – sage (56 records)	Sore throats
Aloe vera – aloe (48 records)	Skin ailments
Solanum tuberosum – potato (47 records)	Burns; Warts
Zingiber officinale – Ginger (37 records)	Stomach problems
Rubus idaeus – Raspberry (37 records)	Childbirth
Sempervivum tectorum – Houseleek (31 records)	Burns; Sore eyes
Vicia faba – Broad Bean (27 records)	Warts
Petroselinum crispum – Parsley (26 records)	Breath freshener

with descriptions of their medicinal uses as well as narratives from British Asians on how their families have used them.

We can therefore see how ethnosciences have been deployed in Britain as a specific means to document, organise and archive for posterity the kind of information about the medicinal uses of plants that is otherwise seen as being at risk, its loss seen as yet another side effect of globalisation and modernisation processes. These ethnosciences have relied on a range of methodologies which all have in common the targeting of peoples' everyday ideas, beliefs, memories and wisdom. This task has been cast as an urgent rescue mission that, for every day that passes, is becoming more and more pressing. Informal herbal medicine use has become a national resource which a number of researchers and projects are now actively trying to chart out and document. Old wives' tales have been transformed into oral histories.

Conclusion: Modernisation and its Side Effects

It was the philosopher Michel Foucault who once argued that the 'blackmail' of the Enlightenment has led to a rather dichotomised impasse: you are either 'for' or 'against' it; 'you either accept the Enlightenment and remain within the tradition of its rationalism, or else you criticize the Enlightenment and then try to escape from its principles of rationality' (Foucault 1997: 313). Perhaps this is Western herbal medicine's dilemma today. On the one hand, there can be no question that if there has been a late-twentieth-century herbal medicine revival in the United Kingdom, as is often claimed, then this revival has in large part been facilitated by the formalisation of its practice, the modernisation of its production and not least the rationalisation of its use. As pointed out earlier, for some this has been a necessary adjustment to the comprehensive social transformations that have occurred in the U.K. following two centuries of urbanisation, industrialisation and more recently globalisation. Yet for others, these developments are a cause for deep concern, especially if they lead towards a 'reductionist' and 'dehumanised' form of herbal medicine where herbs become 'mere' pills to be taken as quick fixes.

Some might argue that a way to bypass this formalisation and rationalisation is to go 'back to the roots' of herbal medicine and seek out and rescue the 'original' country remedies and folk recipes that have been used for centuries by rural people in particular. Yet we must as a minimum ask ourselves whether such a project to rescue folk remedies can avoid the blackmail of the Enlightenment. For, is not the effort to meticulously and systematically document domestic medicine using ethnomethodologies itself contributing to its disciplining and rationalisation? Is it possible to 'merely' document when such knowledge is, for example, to be incorporated into pharmacological research into the active ingredients of some of the most commonly used medicinal plants? And what of those practitioners and users of herbal medicine who resist efforts to formalise and rationalise it? Are they to be seen as hindrances to inevitable progress or as persons with genuine concerns about the directions that herbal medicine is taking in the U.K.? These are the kinds of challenging questions that are being debated today, by herbal practitioners, regulators as well as lay users of herbal medicines, and we can be sure that the dilemmas of modernisation are unlikely to be entirely resolved any time soon.

What I have, nevertheless, shown in this chapter is how the late-twentieth-century revival of herbal medicine is perhaps more accurately accounted for and described as a reinvention of herbal medicine. Today's herbal medicine is certainly not that of Culpeper's or Coffin's day. Not only is herbal medicine practised and used today in an entirely different socio-economic and epidemiological context it is also subject to globalising forces and influences from other traditions of herbal medicine to a much greater extent. As a result, indigenous herbal medicine in Britain has recast itself as 'Western herbal medicine'. Even if this term has by now lost much of its salience due to various global influences, it nevertheless remains in use as a way to distinguish it from Chinese, Ayurvedic or Tibetan herbal medicine. This reinvention has not so much been some kind of ideological shift. Rather, it is best described in terms of its mundanity, in the various practices of formalisation (such as moves towards statutory recognition), rationalisation (such as the transformation of herbals to pharmacopoeias) and documentation (such as the ethnobotanic efforts to chart domestic medicine in the U.K.) that have made it possible.

Notes

1. See, e.g., the two epigraphs which open this chapter. The first comes from an elderly man from Liverpool, and was taken from the Ethnomedica (1999). The second comes from a person from Bradford, and is taken from Plant Cultures (2007).
2. I owe this term to Sue Evans, herbalist and lecturer in herbal medicine at the Southern Cross University who informs me that the phrase is often used in reflexive discussions amongst herbalists in Australia concerning how to be an 'urban herbalist'. The term refers to the alcoholic extracts of plants which are often stored in and dispensed from dark glass bottles. I am also grateful to Nina Nissen for pointing out that in the United Kingdom many urban medical herbalists would certainly not consider themselves a 'black-bottle herbalist' and indeed they often specifically distinguish themselves from those 'phytotherapists' who might rely on such extracts. See more on this issue below.
3. For example, Barbara Griggs's classic was originally sub-titled 'a history of herbal medicine' in 1981 but by its 3rd edition this had been changed to 'the

history and evolution of Western herbal medicine' (Griggs 1997). See also Holmes (1989), which was one of the first published works to distinguish between Western and Chinese herbal medicine in this way. 'Western herbal medicine' often refers to that form which is practiced in North America, the U.K., Australia and New Zealand, although such a distinction has become increasingly fluid and blurred in recent decades as a result of global influences.

4. Compare this to the preamble of the 1858 Medical Act which states that 'it is expedient that Persons requiring Medical Aid should be enabled to distinguish qualified from unqualified Practitioners'.
5. As Brown points out, this has been to the great frustration of herbalists. Brown cites a past president of the Association, who in 1927 lamented that, 'there have been occasions when depression has seized me, and I have realised how powerful are the forces arrayed against us' (Brown 1985: 86).
6. The College of Practitioners of Phytotherapy was originally named the School of Herbal Medicine, then the College of Herbal Medicine, then the College of Phytotherapy until finally settling on its current name in the mid 1990s. My thanks to Nina Nissen for reminding me of these name changes which in themselves indicate some kind of movement.
7. For indigenous British, Chinese and Ayurvedic herbal practitioners.
8. As was the case in the U.K., the 1965 European Council directive on medicinal products sparked a national review of the regulation of medicines in Germany, eventually leading to the passing of a Second Medicines Act in 1976. In order to ensure that all medicines sold in the German market were in compliance with this new act, the German Federal Institute for Drugs and Medical Devices (BfArM) established fifteen commissions to review available quality, safety and efficacy data, wih Commission E being responsible for the review of herbal medicines.
9. See Timmermann (2001) and Kenny (2002) for discussions of how companies like Madaus, supported by the National Socialist regime, took the lead in researching and industrially developing herbal medicines.

References

Ackerknecht, E.H. 1971. *Medicine and Ethnology: Selected Essays*. Baltimore, MD: Johns Hopkins University Press.

Bachelard, G. 2001. *The Formation of the Scientific Mind*. Manchester: Clinamen Press.

BBC. 2002. 'Herbal Remedies "Could Harm Health"'. Retrieved 19 January 2005 from http://news.bbc.co.uk/1/hi/health/2240546.stm.

BMA.1986. 'Alternative Therapy'. London: British Medical Association.

———. 1993. *Complementary Medicine: New Approaches to Good Practice.* Oxford: Oxford University Press.

BPC. 2004. 'Monograph Development'. Retrieved 4 January 2005 from http://www.pharmacopoeia.org.uk/monographdev.cfm.

Brown, P.S. 1985. 'The Vicissitudes of Herbalism in Late Nineteenth- and Early Twentieth-century Britain. *Medical History* 29(1): 71–92.

Canguilhem, G. 1988. *Ideology and Rationality in the History of the Life Sciences.* Cambridge, MA: MIT Press.

Cant, S. and U. Sharma. 1996. *Complementary and Alternative Medicines Knowledge in Practice.* London: Free Association.

Chevallier, A. 1999. *Hypericum: The Natural Anti-depressant and More.* London: Souvenir.

Coward, R. 1989. *The Whole Truth: The Myth of Alternative Health.* London: Faber.

Department of Health, European Herbal Practitioners Association and the Prince of Wales's Foundation for Integrated Health. 2003. 'Recommendations on the Regulation of Herbal Practitioners in the UK: A Report from the Herbal Medicine Regulatory Working Group'. London: The Prince of Wales's Foundation for Integrated Health.

———. 2004 'Reform of Section 12(1) of the Medicines Act 1968: A Draft Report from the Herbal Medicine Regulatory Working Group'. London: Herbal Medicine Regulatory Working Group.

Ethnomedica. 1999. 'Remembered Remedies: Researching the Herbal Traditions of Britain'. Retrieved 7 March 2006 from: http://www.rbgkew.org.uk/ethnomedica/.

European Parliament. 2004. 'Directive 2004/24/EC of the European Parliament and of the Council of 31 March 2004, Amending, as Regards Traditional Herbal Medicinal Products, Directive 2001/83/EC on the Community Code Relating to Medicinal Products for Human Use', *Official Journal of the European Union*, L 136: 85–90.

Foucault, M. 1997. 'What is Enlightenment?' in P. Rabinow (ed.) *Ethics: Subjectivity and Truth.* New York: New Press.

Gaedcke, F. and B. Steinhoff. 2002. *Herbal Medicinal Products.* Washington, DC: CRC Press.

Grieve, M. and C.F. Leyel. 1931. *A Modern Herbal: The Medicinal, Culinary, Cosmetic And Economic Properties, Cultivation And Folk-Lore Of Herbs, Grasses, Fungi, Shrubs, and Trees With All Their Modern Scientific Uses.* New York: Harcourt.

Griggs, B. 1997. *New Green Pharmacy: The Story of Western Herbal Medicine.* London: Vermilion.

Hatfield, G. 2005. *Memory, Wisdom and Healing: The History of Domestic Plant Medicine.* Stroud: Sutton Publishing.

Holmes, P. 1989. *The Energetics of Western Herbs: Integrating Western and Oriental Herbal Medicine Traditions*. Boulder, CO: Artemis Press.

House of Lords. 2000. 'Complementary and Alternative Medicine', report of the Select Committee on Science and Technology. HL Paper 123. London: HMSO.

Illich, I. 1976. *Limits to Medicine: Medical Nemesis and the Expropriation of Health*. London: Boyars.

Jackson-Main, P. 2005. 'Western Herbal Medicine – Gender, Culture and Orthodoxy', in C. O'Sullivan (ed.) *Reshaping Herbal Medicine: Knowledge, Education and Professional Culture*. London: Elsevier.

Jagtenberg, T. and S. Evans. 2003. 'Global Herbal Medicine: A Critique', *Journal of Alternative and Complementary Medicine* 9(2): 321–29.

Kenny, M.G. 2002. 'A Darker Shade of Green: Medical Botany, Homeopathy, and Cultural Politics in Interwar Germany', *Social History of Medicine* 15(3): 481–504.

Larkin, G. 1992. 'Orthodox and Osteopathic Medicine in the Inter-War Years', in M.P. Saks (ed.) *Alternative Medicine in Britain*. Oxford: Clarendon Press.

Malinowski, B. 1922. *Argonauts of the Western Pacific*. London: Routledge and Kegan Paul.

Mills, S. 1993. *The Essential Book of Herbal Medicine*. London: Arkana.

NIMH 1979. 'Memorandum of Association of the National Institute of Medical Herbalists Ltd.' London: NIMH.

______. 2004. 'Herbal Medicine Awareness Week 3-10 September 2004'. Retrieved 19 January 2005 from: http://www.nimh.org.uk/hmaw 04_press.html.

______. 2007. 'A Potted History of Herbal Medicine'. Retrieved 12 July 2007 from: http://www.nimh.org.uk/history.html.

Norris, T. 2004. *Making Sense of Herbal Remedies*. London: Mind.

O'Connor, B.B. 1995. *Healing Traditions: Alternative Medicine and the Health Professions*. Philadelphia: University of Pennsylvania Press.

O'Sullivan, C. (ed.) 2005. *Reshaping Herbal Medicine: Knowledge, Education and Professional Culture*. London: Elsevier.

Plant Cultures. 2007. 'Exploring Plants and People'. Retrieved 8 August 2007 from http://www.plantcultures.org/about.html.

Revill, J. 2005. 'Traditional Remedies Given New Lease of Life as Science Hunts For Fresh Cures', *Observer*, 21 August 2005.

Richter, R.K. 2003. *Herbal Medicine: Chaos in the Marketplace*. New York: Haworth Herbal Press.

Rivers, W.H.R. 1924. *Medicine, Magic and Religion*. London: Kegan Paul, Trench, Trubner.

Saks, M.P. 1992. *Alternative Medicine in Britain*. Oxford: Clarendon Press.

———. 2003. *Orthodox and Alternative Medicine*. London: Sage.

Scottish School of Herbal Medicine. 2006. 'Professional Training in Medical Herbalism'. Retrieved 16 September 2006 from: http://www.herbalmedicine.org.uk/rootpages/yearzero.shtml.

Sharma, U. 1992. *Complementary Medicine Today: Practitioners and Patients*. London: Routledge.

Szerszynski, B. 2005. *Nature, Technology and the Sacred*. Oxford: Blackwell.

Timmermann, C. 2001. 'Rationalizing "folk medicine" in Interwar Germany: Faith, Business, and Science at "Dr. Madaus & Co."', *Social History of Medicine* 14(3): 459–82.

Wahlberg, A. 2007a. 'Measuring Progress: Calculating the Life of Nations'. *Distinktion: Scandinavian Journal of Social Theory* 14: 65–82.

———. 2007b. 'A Quackery with a Difference: New Medical Pluralism and the Problem of "Dangerous Practitioners" in the United Kingdom', *Social Science and Medicine* 65: 2307–16.

———. 2008a. 'Above and Beyond Superstition: Western Herbal Medicine and the Decriminalising of Placebo', *History of the Human Sciences* 21(1): 77–101.

———. 2008b. 'Pathways to Plausibility: When Herbs become Pills', *BioSocieties* 3(1): 37–56.

Chapter 7

Crystal and Spiritual Healing in Northern England: Folk-inspired Systems of Medicine

Stuart McClean

Introduction

The World Health Organisation has claimed that people living in non-Western or 'developing' societies receive the majority of their health care from indigenous or 'traditional' medicine (WHO 2002). In such societies, drawing a demarcation between orthodox as opposed to 'folk' or heterodox medicine is unlikely to be meaningful. In common perhaps with Britain prior to the latter part of the nineteenth century, some of these societies have held to a plural system of healthcare. With the widespread proliferation of complementary and alternative medicine (CAM) one could argue that the situation in many of these societies is not completely dissimilar to the one we are witness to in Britain today; superficially at least there is a notable return to a form of medical pluralism. Moreover, despite the increased attention to questions of regulation, formalisation and professionalisation, many complementary health practitioners still depend on their practices' received 'folk' wisdom, and many adhere to the principles that are central to folk healing.

In this chapter I consider the significance and meaning of contemporary folk healing, in the form of crystal and spiritual healing practices.[1] In England, spiritual healing has its roots in spiritualism and the spiritualist practices of Victorian society prevalent between the 1860s and 1880s, the proverbial 'golden age' of spiritualism

(Owen 2004).[2] During the mid Victorian period, and at a time of a perceived crisis of faith (Oppenheim 1985), England fostered a significant social and historical tradition of religious and 'spiritualist' healing – such as Mesmerism – with its origins in the north and north-east of England (Barrow 1986; Owen 2004). Such heterodox 'spiritualist' and spiritual healing practices, inclusive of Pentecostalism and Christian Science, were also prevalent in the United States during this time (Lee 1976; Braude 1989; English-Lueck 1990). Evidenced in spiritualist approaches such as mediumship, they are based on the idea that entering a state of 'trance' allows the individual a form of communication between the living and the dead and empirical proof of the immortality of the soul. These practices were deemed spiritually meaningful by their proponents, though they also reflected materialist – social and scientific – concerns of the Victorian age (Braude 1989; Owen 2004).[3]

Here I consider the revitalisation and reinvention of these folk-inspired spiritual practices, but with features that are new to the contemporary scene. One such practice is crystal healing, best described as a 'fringe' and esoteric therapy used in conjunction with other spiritual healing practices, particularly those deemed 'New Age'.[4] CAM practices such as crystal and spiritual healing are commonly practised by individuals and at healing centres that exert little regulatory control over their practices, and the case discussed in this chapter is no exception to this. The status of crystal healing as one of the more minor or 'fringe' complementary health practices is further confirmed by its place in a major House of Lords Select Committee review of complementary medicine (House of Lords 2000).

This chapter reports on ethnographic research carried out in the late 1990s, which explored healing practices and practitioners at an institutional centre for healing in the north of England. The Centre was founded and run by a charismatic and entrepreneurial healer, whilst other healers used the Centre to practice and share knowledge. Folk healing practices are infrequently associated with such organised institutions, but one of the key philosophies which emerged at the Centre was to do with encouraging healers to locate and establish their own unique, individualised practice, 'what works for you'. The healers thus practised personalised systems of healing, which were in turn sanctioned by the institutional philosophy of the healing Centre and its founder. This situation can be seen as particularly paradoxical, and it also raises important questions about the boundaries between folk healing knowledge and more systematised and culturally legitimate forms of CAM. This chapter also alludes to the impact of professionalisation processes, such as training and other forms of systematisation, on healing practices with folk origins.

Crystal and Spiritual Healing

Crystals, amulets and gemstones have been used as healing objects, as well as for protection, decoration and adornment, in a range of cultural and healing traditions across the world.[5] Social scientists exploring both the New Age phenomenon and the growth of CAM have tended to see crystal healing as typical of an emerging New Age movement (Sharma 1992; Hess 1993; Brown 1997). Within this schema, crystal healing, or the 'laying-on of stones', has been widely perceived by observers as the middle-class New Age healing activity par excellence. Moreover, crystal healers, even amongst complementary therapists, have earned themselves a dubious reputation. Amongst the medical profession and the media things are worse, and as peddlers of 'gobbledygook' (Sample 2007), they are placed as rather marginal and insignificant complementary therapists amongst the gamut of available CAM.[6]

Too much attention in the existing research, however, had been given over to generalising the phenomenon by relying on 'expert' New Age writers, making broad statements about a 'movement', and neglecting the issue of local variation and atypical cases. Crystal and spiritual healing as practice and as ideology (its culturally situated meaningfulness) needs to be understood in the contexts in which it emerges and is practised. As Napolitano and Flores explain in their analysis of CAM practices in Mexico: 'alternative and "traditional" forms of medical knowledge cannot be disentangled from those who practise them: knowledge cannot be disembodied, nor de-contextualized from its strategic applications. It is always a form of situated knowledge' (Napolitano and Flores 2003: 82).

Hands-on spiritual healing also featured prominently during my fieldwork. Hands-on healing, or what is also referred to as the 'laying-on of hands', is an established and indeed increasingly ubiquitous tradition in healing communities. Hands-on healing is synonymous with the healing activities of Christian groups, metaphysical and psychic healers, and mediumistic and spiritual healers (see Skultans 1974; Benor 1984; Easthope 1986; McGuire 1988; Frohock 1992). In Western societies, crystal healing is used predominantly by spiritual healers of a New Age persuasion, both as an adjunct to hands-on healing and as a healing practice in its own right. Such practices constitute 'symbolic healing systems' (Glik 1988) in that their effect and power relies on the ritualised, metaphorical and mimetic nature of their actions.

Folk healing, if there is a definition free of ambiguity, refers to healing practices that are historically situated and rooted, non-systematised, and learned informally – perhaps through word of mouth or through a loose and open 'system' of apprenticeship – and draw on direct experience, though the boundaries between folk healing and CAM are fluid and contextual. In this chapter, by evoking a particular ethnographic context, I identify aspects of contemporary crystal and spiritual healing that typically exemplify folk healing in some ways, but in other ways raise important questions and dilemmas about the boundaries (both metaphorical and concrete) between the folk and the mainstream, as well as the boundaries between folk healing and CAM.

The Ethnographic Context: The Vital Energy Healing Centre

The fieldwork for the ethnographic study took place in a town in the north of England not particularly renowned for alternative therapies, though it is not drastically untypical of other contexts where New Age healing flourishes. The Vital Energy Healing Centre (VEHC) was a short walk from the centre of the town.[7] Other retail shops in close proximity to the healing centre included a trophy shop, a fish and chip shop and a carpet salesroom. From the outside, the healing centre looked inconspicuous: a three storey Victorian terraced house, the only visible sign marking it off as different to the other shops and dwellings being a small placard above the door giving the name of the business, decorated brightly in all the colours of the rainbow. Inside was a different story: a veritable Aladdin's Cave of brightly coloured murals and posters with New Age depictions of religious and mythical figures as well as dolphins. Crystals of all shapes, sizes and colours were laid out haphazardly in the reception area of the Centre on the ground floor, taking up most of the available space, although there was also room for a desk, some chairs for visitors and clients, as well as other gift-type objects, such as greeting cards, dream catchers, joss sticks and aromatherapy bottles.

One of the healing rooms, known as the 'front room', was located on the ground floor. On the first floor were two more healing rooms: one was called the 'sanctuary', a room that acted as the focal point for group meditation every Wednesday evening; the other, across the landing on the first floor, was the 'pink room'. On the second floor was an office, in the process of renovation, as well as a guest room cum library, which contained a vast range of esoteric and mystical texts. The 'front room' and the 'pink room' contained a biomedical-style couch for clients to lie on during healing; rolls of Kimberly Clark paper towels were fixed to the wall. A small hand basin was located in the corner of the 'front room'. This was not used for washing or sterilising medical equipment, but for 'cleansing and purifying' the healing crystals. The presence and use of flowers, candles, joss sticks, New Age type paintings of Jesus and other religious figures, all denoted a curious, eclectic fusion of medicine, healing and a broad, syncretic religiosity.

The owner and principal healer at the Centre, Teresa, established the business in 1981. Teresa organised the business side of the Centre as well as teaching crystal healing as part of a diploma-level crystal-healing course. She was also active in the establishment of national standards through her participation in a national healing organisation. As Teresa taught healers that subsequently set up their own healing Centres, she oversaw their activities on behalf of this quasi-regulatory body. In this respect, the healing Centre was closer to the activities and philosophy of complementary medicine than folk healing. In addition to the training programme, Teresa oversaw other healers who used the rooms at the Centre for a percentage of their earnings. Teresa's project at the Centre in many ways mirrored the professionalisation process that many healing Centres have undergone in order to widen their appeal and safeguard their practices.

The healers at the Centre charged a fee for their healing services, which again is atypical of folk healing, although they all operated sliding fee scales as well as providing free sessions and forms of gift exchange. One client who attended the centre regularly would give vegetables and flowers from his allotment in exchange for healing; such non-economic exchanges were regular amongst a local community which was not particularly wealthy. Such systems of exchange are also more common with folk healers as opposed to complementary medicine practitioners.

In addition to healing sessions and workshops, Teresa attended to her crystal-healing course, which she set up in response to the interest crystal healing had received over the years; much of this interest stemmed from ex-clients. This is significant because through a period of treatment clients are often encouraged to discover healing ability in themselves (the 'gift'). This is no surprise, as a key healing tenet at the centre was the notion that the client holds important individual (and expert) knowledge about their own body. An emphasis on the 'personalisation' in New Age forms of folk healing stands in sharp contrast to the 'depersonalisation' evident in formal biomedicine.

The Route to Healing Identities: Identifying the 'Gift' and the Calling

The healers I encountered at the Centre, Teresa notwithstanding, talked about the ways that they got involved in healing. Each of their stories was unique but there were common themes that linked together their individual narratives. Charlie, for instance, was a young male healer, and a local person, in his late twenties. The healers that I had spoken to at the centre by the time I met Charlie were all women. Apart from one other, older male healer, Charlie was the only male healer who played a key role in the life of the Centre. Charlie was a bodybuilder as well as a healer.

Before attending the Centre as a client, Charlie was reliant on the use of steroids to build his muscles for lifting weights, which led to both physical and emotional difficulties. In order to counteract the pain that the steroids were causing he took painkillers. Charlie explained, 'I was in a real mess', and added; 'I'm now going to look at how crystals can help me in weight training, you know, doing it the natural way'. Charlie also claimed that there was a genuine physical reason for the healing interest: 'Before I started coming here I used to feel my hands burning up all the time, like they were on fire. When I came here and asked Teresa what it was that I was feeling, she said it was because I was a healer and have also been a healer in my past lives'.

In common with many of the healers at the Centre, the underlying issue here is that Charlie visited a healer in connection with some ill health and/or emotional, psychosocial problems. His visit to a healer was prompted by his growing addiction to steroid drugs for bodybuilding. His realisation about his healing potential, encouraged by the other healers at the Centre, gave him another chance and allowed him to channel his energies into a new venture, albeit one that was significantly different to bodybuilding. There are issues that also resonate with the folk healing literature, particularly surrounding the initiation into healing circles and that healers experience the sensation, not always unpleasant, of heat through the hands (see Snow 1978; Hufford 1988; Alver 1995). For Charlie, the experience of being brought into healing symbolises the 'calling', one which is brought on by other healers recognising the 'gift' of the ability to channel healing energy.

As a healer with a perceived 'gift', Charlie seemed critical of Teresa's attempts to professionalise and standardise activities at the Centre. On the occasion that such issues were discussed by Teresa and the other healers, Charlie expressed open hostility to these agendas. Charlie believed in doing his own thing, manifested in both his healing practice and in his critical attitude towards Teresa's vested interest in professionalism. Such blatant individualism, exemplified by Charlie, was allowable as the 'folk' philosophy of the Centre – 'what works for you' – sanctioned this approach. For example, on one occasion Teresa proudly informed me that the Centre was setting up a crystal-healing diploma that would run in conjunction with a complementary medicine course at a university in the Midlands. Charlie was singularly unimpressed and pulled a disgruntled face: 'Part of a university degree, eh? Oh yeah, right!' His response showed significant opposition towards Teresa's approaches and its inherent professionalisation agenda.

The two other healers that I came into the most contact with over the fieldwork period were Stella and Sally, both women in their fifties. Stella had been practising hands-on healing for approximately eight years. Like Charlie, Stella ventured into healing after visiting the Centre as a client. Stella experienced a form of lower back pain (osteoarthritis) for many years and biomedical treatment could only treat the symptoms. As she explained: 'I was told I had osteoarthritis and the GP said that I had to go and learn to live with it. Now, I wasn't going to do that, I'm not like that. So, I started coming here and seeing Teresa, which helped, and then I became a healer. I started with crystals and then later learned hypnotherapy'. Although primarily a hands-on spiritual healer, Stella also practised crystal healing. Much of her free time was spent at the Centre's open and free healing session on a Wednesday evening, referred to as 'meditation night'.

Sally was also an established and valued member of the Centre. A longstanding friend of Teresa, Sally offered her healing services free of charge at the Centre on Wednesday evenings. By day she was employed locally at a residential care home which became the source of a number of problems. Like many of the healers I came into contact with, Sally took pleasure in looking after those around her, but over two years of employment at the care home the work had drained her both physically and emotionally. Teresa explained that the frequent physical illness Sally experienced came about because she got too involved in patients' lives. For example, on meditation night Sally normally asked Teresa to 'send out' healing energy to her patients at the care home ('absent' or 'distant' healing also featured prominently at the Centre).

One day Sally came into the Centre visibly upset. Five patients at the care home, whom Sally had become attached to, had died over the space of a few weeks. Whilst Teresa admired Sally's compassion, she felt that she should retain more distance from the patients, as this could affect her health: 'The problem is, Sally gets too emotionally involved, and they [the care home staff] have told her not to, but Sally will do what she wants. I think they want you to be a compassionate person without being involved'. Indeed, Sally often rang in to say she couldn't heal because she was too tired or not feeling well.

A common issue is that the healer's interest in healing largely developed during their time as a client, a familiar theme in the folk-healing literature. Such a collective of similarly afflicted people in healing groups is not surprising, as 'part of the treatment is to be initiated into a fellowship of the similarly afflicted' (Frankenberg 1986: 621). Edgar, in a social anthropological study of therapeutic 'dreamwork' groups, explains that the participants in his study were often propelled to join the group as a way of reflecting on more general life crises or transitions. As Edgar states, 'Almost all the members who stayed through a group term of ten weeks disclosed either to the group or in the follow-up interviews that they were going through a period of their life which involved, in their eyes, great change or considerable crisis' (Edgar 1995: 10).[8] There are therefore important similarities between healing and the initiation into folk and other shamanic traditions: 'Many of those who were in the process of becoming healers had experienced a dramatic healing or improvement in some condition or illness prior to trying to heal others ... Sickness of the healer prior to initiation is similar to the process of shamanistic initiation in other cultures' (Glik 1988: 1200).[9]

Stella's and Sally's involvement as healers at the Centre is also a consequence of their experiences with formal biomedicine, and it conveys a larger story about the lack of control that people face in the context of their experiences with biomedical treatment. For example, Stella often made allusions to how older people are not treated seriously by the medical profession, and that this attitude impacted on the way she was treated by doctors. As a lay person she did not wield the power and autonomy that expert-based knowledge confers upon the individual. As a consequence, her healing practices and ideas, not unlike other healers at the Centre, manifested themselves as a unique combination of the spiritual approach and folk-inspired common-sense ones.

The Personalised and Individuated Nature of Healing Practice

Teresa's role as head of the Centre was partly to enforce the primary ideological premise: healers are encouraged to practice their form of crystal healing, a premise quite unlike many CAM therapies. Individuation – or the creative act or will to express individuality – was a central philosophy at the Centre, and expressing agency or being individual was institutionalised at the Centre as a form of collective ideology. One consequence of this extreme personalisation and individuation was that crystal and spiritual healing enabled the healer to develop their own distinctive style of healing. Crucially, this individuation provided its own legitimacy (which here I term 'internal' legitimacy), and represented a move away from the kind of legitimacy conferred by science, medicine and/or community ('external' legitimacy).

For the healers, individuation denoted three things. First, healers recognised and celebrated the individually constructed nature of health, illness and disease. Second, healers (and clients) created, adopted and utilised healing practices and diagnostic procedures that were also individually constructed. Finally, their understanding of health, the body and illness also manifested themselves in individual and highly personalised theories. The emphasis on individuation, I suggest, is particularly prevalent in a form of CAM like crystal healing, because it engages with spirituality and celebrates, at its core, folk notions about the body, health and illness. Let us now turn to some examples of how such personalisation worked in practice, and consider what this reveals about the folk-inspired nature of such healing practices.

'Good Vibrations': The Nature of Health and Illness, and How Healing Works

One area that personalisation clearly operated in is healers' explanations of the healing process, and in particular the concept of intuition in healing diagnosis. However, first let us consider how healers conceptualise health and illness. Healers at the Centre perceived health not as the absence of disease but as the absence of 'blockages' that occur first in the 'chakra' or 'etheric' areas of the body. Chakras are defined as the area where 'vital' energy in the etheric or spiritual body intersects with an area in the physical or material body. The blockages are seen as being caused by 'negativity' and negative emotions, which may arise from the individual themselves or from an external agent. As individuals we therefore have a moral responsibility to protect ourselves from these negative energies (see McClean 2005 for a fuller description of this process). As Teresa explained: 'You see, a lot of our illnesses are caused by personal, private problems. It's those emotions that block our chakras and cloud our auras'. Such blockages are removed either by the hands of the healer or by a crystal that is able to act as a 'scalpel', drawing the negative energies out. The healer may employ a number of techniques to ensure protection of their own spiritual bodies, a method that bore more than a passing resemblance to other folk-healing practices (see Fisch 1968).

Hufford (1988) has suggested that a common feature of folk healing is the focus on 'energy', which connects folk traditions of healing to the theory of 'vitalism', also prominent in New Age healing. Healers at the Centre saw healing as the process of transferring (and sometimes 'injecting') positive healing energy into the client whilst simultaneously drawing negative energies out of the etheric or spiritual body. For example, healers sometimes used a 'laser-wand' crystal to 'blast' energy into the patient, which at the same time would also draw 'harmful energies' out of the patient's spiritual body. The implications and significance of such mimicry of formal medical practice has been discussed elsewhere (McClean 2003). Hufford's description of a Pennsylvanian Pow-wow healer's practice has obvious parallels with the healers' approach at the VEHC, as well as Mexican-American *curanderos*: 'Folk healers often view their activities as based on a transfer of good energies into the patient and the removal of negative forces from him' (Hufford 1988: 239). In his discussion of Norwegian folk healers, Alver also recounts a similar process in which a healer with warm hands can 'heal by dissolving "blockages" in the body through "radiation" from the palms of his hands' (Alver 1995: 27).

The practice of crystal and spiritual healing represents a continuing trend with what is thus termed 'energy medicine', of which there are folk and 'professional' variations. Nevertheless, energy is seen as a shared concept amongst CAM therapists (see, e.g., McGuire 1988; Frohock 1992; O'Connor 2000; Fadlon 2004), although it is more commonly associated with New Age practices (English-Lueck 1990). More specifically, the New Age healers' focus on concepts such as 'energy' or 'vital force' represents a clear challenge to the scientific concept of the body as machine (Synnott 1992; O'Connor 1995).

A similar term used is 'vibrational healing' and refers to that which is beyond the material. The concept implies that behind the spiritual engagement with healing is a physical process; the term 'vibrational' denotes physical changes. In healing, the term refers to spiritual-level changes, although I stress that there is some overlap, as it is argued that healing that takes place at the spiritual level impacts on the physical body at a later stage. There are notable similarities between the concept of vibration in healing (Gerber 2001) and that of 'pulsation' which is more commonly used in Buddhist and Hindu thought (Singh 1992). In the following section I highlight how something as individual and personalised as the senses is central to the perceived success of healing energies.

The Senses in 'Vibrational' Healing

On one occasion Teresa explained the concept of 'resonance' to a group of healing trainees (myself included) in the sanctuary. She came into the room laden with an assortment of brass-coloured bowls and wooden pestles. Each of the bowls was individually made, had different markings, and was made of a composite of seven metals: lead, mercury, copper, nickel, silver, gold and brass. She also showed us a chime-type instrument that she struck with a crystal to give us some idea of the different sounds.

As Teresa chimed the instrument, she asked the healing trainees to 'feel' where the sound resonated in the body. Two trainees – Adele and Helen – closed their eyes to feel the sounds more clearly. Teresa then explained how the chiming bowls and other calming sounds can change the 'atmosphere' of a room, as sound alters the vibrations of an environment. She argued that sound can also alter the vibration of an individual, as it is used to bring 'clarity' to the chakras. As such, the bowls should be used before healing or personal meditation. As Teresa explained 'The sound can be used to balance and cleanse the chakras. You should hold them [the bowls] under the base with the palm of your hand, and press the wooden stick against the rim, moving it at a constant speed around the bowl. With the chime I also use crystals to tap the keys to make a sound, as I think that with the crystals you get a clearer sound'.

On another occasion Teresa asked us to explore the sense of smell, again using the 'resonance' technique. Taking each of the healing trainees in turn, she demonstrated channelling an 'essential oil' (aromatherapy oil) through the hands and asked us how we experienced the vibration of the oils. This was achieved by the healer rubbing the oil onto their own hands and wafting the smell over the client's aura. Teresa went on to suggest that the vibration of a crystal, flower or oil can be channelled or resonate through anything because it doesn't matter what physical barriers exist. 'With the energy of vibration you can get through anything: concrete, wood, glass, whatever', she said.

The senses clearly play a key role in vibrational healing. It is argued by healers that vibrational healing operates at a level beyond the physical. Rendering physical barriers obsolete, vibrational healing operates on a 'subtle' level of healing energy. For a healer to 'tune in' they must, it is claimed, raise the level of their senses and become 'sensitive' to the healing process. The healer's emphasis on the senses highlights the folk-inspired (as well as feminised) nature of crystal healing as it is healers with the 'gift' for being 'sensitive' that are better able to 'tune in' to healing energies.[10]

The Crystals and the Stones: Not Just Any Old Rock

Drifting around New Age shops and other related premises that sell crystals, as I frequently did during my fieldwork period, it was interesting to note how many people purchased crystals as 'lucky charms', such as amulets, all imbued with powerful personal meaning. Whilst sitting in the reception area of the Centre reading a book or engaged in conversation with healers or clients, I was able to watch people come and go, pick up crystals, feel them in their hands, taking note of the colour, shape, clarity and so on. People browsing in reception were often just passers-by, perhaps purchasing a crystal for a friend or a relative. Most importantly, they would ask one of us what 'something was good for', hoping for the perfect crystal for their problem, a strategy not unlike that of many other folk remedies, like the copper bracelet.

Crystals embody particular qualities that can be isolated and looked up in a crystal healing textbook. Crystal healers frequently refer to these textbook typologies of crystals when making decisions about which crystals to use in healing, but other healers were more prepared to make their own decisions rather than follow those of the experts in the textbooks, thus making their own intuitive and individual choices over crystal selection. Jenny, a healer who was taught by Teresa but worked in a neighbouring town, said: 'Often the properties in the books for each stone are all vastly different, so you have to go by what you think. There are guidelines with the colours of the chakras though … the chakras are divided by colour, although you can place a crystal from one area into another if it feels right'. The general guiding principle – 'if it feels right' – reflects the idea that healing is individuated rather than systematised and expert-based.

In addition, one of the ways in which healing beliefs or practices can be defined as 'folk' is by considering its indigenous application. Geographically, folk concepts and constructs are frequently bounded by symbolic constructions of space and place. Here, healers provided their own version of this geographically-bounded construct particularly when considering the significance of which crystals to use and whether the energies of crystals differed depending on where they were sourced. As rocks, crystals are said to represent indigenous healing energies. Quartz is found widely in all parts of the world and the U.K. is no exception. Teresa stressed the importance in using crystals indigenous to your area. This was reflected in an occasion when Teresa handed round some Blue John stone to assist in a group meditation. A stone indigenous to the Derbyshire Peak District in the U.K., Teresa felt that the use of Blue John would intensify the meditation experience. After our meditation and group reflection, Teresa added: 'These are indigenous stones of course, they are hand gathered, and with this comes a purer experience in meditation'. As natural objects they are rooted in the healer's idea about what constitutes a natural environment. Teresa's concern for rooting the experience of healing in local contexts is also symbolic of crystal healing's folk origins.

Informal Knowledge Transmission and Learning in Crystal Healing

In exploring contemporary 'New Age' crystal and spiritual healing, and the boundaries between 'folk' and CAM, the final theme I want to consider is that of healing-knowledge transmission, socialisation and learning. Along with six other novice healers, I attended the crystal healing diploma at the VEHC. Teresa and I agreed that in order for me to carry out my research on healing effectively I would have to take part in a training course for a diploma in crystal healing. Attending the diploma training provided me with some important insights into the process of becoming a healer, and it offered me legitimate access to other curative practices. I also attended partly in response to other healers at the Centre who said that I should get more involved.

The diploma course was loosely structured and addressed topics and themes which were considered central to crystal healing. However, despite some systematised and professionalised elements the course relied mostly on exploring intuitive knowledge and encouraging healers to develop their own healing style. The diploma was taught in two-day blocks, six times per year over two years, and at the end of the course healer apprentices had to write a lengthier dissertation-type study about an aspect of their practice and its relationship to 'theory'. The teaching on the course itself was unstructured; most sessions emphasised the importance and value of the individual's knowledge over that of a book or so-called 'expert'. In the following I provide a description of two illustrative examples from my fieldwork about the process of learning crystal-healing knowledge and being a healing apprentice.

Crystal Healing: Example A

On this occasion the crystal healing apprentices, myself included, were upstairs in the sanctuary with Teresa. Teresa wrote the following on the whiteboard:

> Resonance Therapy
> Everything resonates at a different rate
> Everything *has* a vibration

She then explained how the flow of energy can transfer from the resonating object to what she called the 'generator' (the healer's hand). Here, Teresa demonstrated one of her styles of crystal healing called 'resonance therapy'. The purpose of resonance therapy is to enable the patient to maintain a semi-alert state of mind, so that the healer can carry out 'deep work'. Out of our group of apprentices

(Elsie, Sarah, Margaret, Anne, Katie and I), Sarah volunteered and got on the couch. Teresa then explained the healing:

> When you are healing somebody it is important to use visualisations when you can. These can be guided visualisations in that you can take the patient through it and this helps the patient to release anything that is inside them. I think it is important for you to develop your own kind of guided visualisation. Try to vary it as well from time to time, depending of course on what you want to open the patient up to.

Teresa started the healing session and described her actions as she progressed. 'You should place – as you know – one clear quartz at the feet pointing up, one at the crown pointing down and one in each of the palms of the hands'. She asked Sarah whether she was left-handed, which she wasn't. 'First, you ask for guidance, and then you ask for a blessing for your healing'. She grasped her crystal pendulum and moved it nonchalantly over each chakra point, remarking that as it swings wildly you take that as a sign of an imbalanced chakra, 'You balance each chakra as you move the pendulum down the body. The pendulum will go from spinning fast and with a wide arc, to circling slowly. Once the pendulum reaches the feet so as to check the "earth star", it can be moved up again through each of the chakra points to check that they have been balanced okay'.

Teresa then explained that she was going to 'channel' the energy of a 'tumbled' turquoise crystal.[11] The energy of the turquoise was channelled through Teresa's body (from the left arm), over the head, down the right arm and out of the right hand. With her hand above the 'soul star', she said that light would usher in at this chakra point.[12] She moved on to the crown chakra, then the brow, each time asking Sarah questions related to the sensations she experienced. She used open questions such as: 'Where would you like to go with [such and such a colour]?'; 'What do you want to do with that sensation?'; and 'What are you feeling with this energy?' However, she said the questions should never be too specific: 'Counselling is not giving advice. It's letting them go with what they are experiencing'. Furthermore,

> You need to question the patients very gently, to ask them what they are experiencing. Whether, if they see a golden light, they want to wrap themselves in it or breathe it in, or anything else. This is very important. Also, they may experience visualising pictures, memories of their childhood

> or a painful memory. If you find that you have hit on a difficult memory then you can leave it if they don't really want to explore it, and then you can return to it at a later stage if you can take a note of it. You should ask them what they want to do with the picture or the memory or the object or whatever, and don't forget to do that. You are the instrument and you should fine tune the instrument for what you are doing, whatever the purpose of the healing is.

At the brow chakra, Teresa explained, 'It is important to give them plenty of space at the brow chakra. Don't press too heavily'. She held the crystal about six inches above Sarah's brow point and asked her if the energy was too strong. It was, so Teresa moved her hand up until Sarah was more comfortable, about twelve inches above the chakra point. Teresa continued, 'That is very important for the three higher chakras, but for the lower chakras you can sometimes find yourself wanting to press right in so that it feels like you are almost touching them'. As Teresa reached the throat chakra, Sarah said she was experiencing a rush of golden light: 'What do you want to do with that light? Do you want to wrap yourself in it?' Teresa asked. 'I am the light', Sarah replied, matter of factly. 'I feel like I am the universe. It's a wonderful feeling', she added. 'Good', said Teresa, 'Stay with the golden light for a while'.

At this stage Teresa's hand shook slightly. She explained later that she received very strong vibrations from the throat and heart chakras. At the end, Teresa said you can place a few drops of oil (she used jasmine) onto the palms of your hands and wave it into the patient's aura, as this establishes calmness after the healing. With the oil in her hands, she moved them around the contours of Sarah's aura, making flat stroking actions as if straightening out a tablecloth. An alternative, she said, is to hold the bottle of the oil in the left hand along with the crystal. The crystal should point into the bottle of oil. This channels the vibration of the oil through the palm of your right hand. She later added that you should not channel more than three things during a healing: the crystal, an oil remedy and a flower would be sufficient.

Crystal Healing: Example B

On this occasion, Jack, a male healer and reflexologist is his late fifties, joined us for the day to teach some healing techniques. The first healing practice Jack demonstrated was the 'aura scan'. We were sat upstairs in the pink room and Jack asked who would like to volunteer. 'Who would like a bit of a boost this morning?' he said merrily. Elsie seemed keen, so she climbed onto the couch. Jack then placed a crystal in the palm of each of her hands, the left one pointing to the heel of the hand and the right one towards the tips of the fingers. The healer holds the same crystals in their own hands in this manner. Jack then went through the invocation with the rest of us, which we repeated together. 'I invoke the light of the Christ within. I am a clear and perfect channel. Light is my guide'.

This was repeated three times. Then he placed his right hand on Elsie's hand and his left hand on her brow. He called this 'bridging', and explained further, 'which hand goes where depends upon which side of the client you are on. If you are on the left side, your left finger would be on the wrist and the right finger on the brow. You will then feel immediately a tingling sensation as the patient's energy field attunes to you and your crystals'.

Jack said that the crystal in the right hand should be placed loosely between the thumb and the fingers with the point towards the thumb. This crystal is then passed through the 'etheric energy field' (the aura) surrounding the body, and scans the body for imbalances. These imbalances, or what are sometimes termed 'blockages', create 'signals' which individuals detect in individually unique ways. As he explained:

> Slowly move the crystal over the body from one side to the other. Now, feel any difference. These differences are signals of problem areas, energy blockages or weaknesses. They may be very subtle. Some detect the sensation as resistance, some as heat. Other people feel it as a sensation of cold. Don't worry if you feel hot and I feel cold. It doesn't then mean that I'm right and you're wrong – we're all individuals. Some people receive these signals fast and their conscious mind can't interpret them. It doesn't matter. They just know there is a blockage at that spot.

Jack pointed out that when a 'signal' is detected, you should stop at that area. At this point he directed the tip of the crystal to the place where he had stopped on Elsie, the right shoulder. He explained that you then circle the crystal from right to left until a strong pulling sensation is felt, drawing the crystal towards the body. He circled the crystal towards Elsie and then touched its tip on her shoulder. He said that this action grounds the change you have been making in the spirit body down to the physical body.

He continued to 'scan', moving down the body, repeating the process each time he picked up on a blocked area. As he moved the crystal down the body he scanned side to side, but explained that you can scan in any direction. Once he reached Elsie's feet he said he was rescanning the body, which is designed to go back and check on any particular areas that you may have missed. He termed this process the 'onion-peel effect'. By this he meant that the layers of suppressed emotions which can surface during healing are removed once the healing is complete.

At the end of the healing session he smoothed out the aura by moving his hands over the body with the crystals in either hand, a process he called 'smoothing the feathers'. This was achieved by moving the crystals with both hands down the body, starting at the head and descending to the feet. Following this Elsie got up off of the couch and the crystals were 'purified' in the basin.

Healing Apprenticeship and the Role of Innovation

In both healing examples we can note that healing is taught as a dynamic between structure (particular techniques, questions and gestures) and improvisation. Occasionally during fieldwork I experienced this dynamic as a tension, and one that was often paradoxical. Healers at the VEHC were encouraged to be creative and innovative and it was clear that the Centre supported and legitimated this creativity. This also gave credence to the notion that healing at the Centre was individuated as opposed to expert-led or systematised. However, there were aspects of these healing practices that could be considered folk-inspired. As exemplified at the VEHC, healing practices were placed on various ends of a spectrum – from the wholly individuated and personalised to the more expert-led and systematised. Along this spectrum are more folk-inspired practices and beliefs, ones which stem from the group and community-led nature of the healing Centre, and which provided the origins for many of their ideas about health and well-being.

Innovation arose initially from the healer's apprenticeship and training, in which they were often encouraged to mimic and draw upon another healer's style and, additionally, bring into play more personalised practices. Furthermore, both the media and the method of learning gave rise to individual innovation. As healing knowledge at the Centre was neither written down nor passed on through intensive study, healing rituals are cursorily learnt from observation and then subjected to unfettered individual interpretation and modification.

I suggest that individuation is codified and sanctioned within the healing Centre as the normal orientation towards healing practice and knowledge. This can be noted in Teresa's suggestion that 'You are the instrument', by which she implied that the healer controls the event and generates the healing power. And yet we can see that there is a sense in which patient 'control' (as well as mutual 'interaction') over the experience of healing is also important, as Teresa had implied in her statement that healers should be 'letting patients go with what they are experiencing'. Personalised expression is therefore 'internally' legitimated through the ideology of the Centre. Again, Jack explained that it is not important if healers detected the 'sensations' at different times or even in the wrong order, because the sensations are 'subtle' and 'we're all individuals'.

Conclusion: Folk Inspired Systems of Medicine

In this chapter I have provided a cursory look into one of the more fringe and marginalised practices of complementary and alternative medicine. Crystal and spiritual healers are clearly attempting to engage in discourses of formalisation and professionalisation, and there were attempts by Teresa to bring more standardisation into the practices of the Vital Energy Healing Centre. However, we can note how healers at the Centre were heavily influenced by and acted upon folk models and conceptualisations of healing. This was evident in their approach to health and illness, as well as being a central part of their overall philosophy of healing and their approach to healing socialisation and the transmission of knowledge.

The healers' general philosophy at the Centre, in which they practised 'what works for you', encouraged a reliance on both individual and personalised knowledge as well as folk-inspired practices and beliefs. In deliberately distancing themselves from the depersonalised nature of formal medicine, this emphasis on individuated knowledge permeated all aspects and activities of the Centre as well as the process whereby one became a healer. Although

Teresa had a clear and vested interest in standardising aspects of healing practice, which can be taken as evidence of dealing with the wider project of professionalising 'folk' knowledge, the other healers maintained a significant distance from this, partly due to their own stories about coming to healing, but also because of the creativity and sense of agency they could achieve through generating their own practices and techniques. The endurance of such 'folk' models was also evident in the endurance of non-monetarised relationships and systems of exchange within the community (see Chapter 11, this volume, for a further discussion of this theme).

We can thus see how the agenda promoted by the House of Lords, the Department of Health, the World Health Organisation and other agencies is unlikely to influence how more spiritual and folk-inspired healing practices operate. Healers as well as their clients are drawn largely to the 'anything goes' philosophy of healing and the Centre, and so are unlikely to engage sufficiently with processes of professionalisation and regulation (despite Teresa's attempts otherwise). Although clearly paradoxical, crystal and spiritual healing, as it is experienced through one particular Centre in the north of England, presents itself as a 'system' of folk healing knowledge and practice; a model of personalised medicine for our postmodern times.

Notes

1. This chapter draws upon and reproduces some previously published material and data, with permission of the Edwin Mellen Press (see McClean 2006).
2. 'Spiritualist' is the name given to individuals interested in all aspects of the spiritual (not just healing), and although not a religion in the conventional sense, these practices are frequently tied to the activities of spiritualist churches.
3. A key theme in both Braude's (1989) writing on the United States and Owen's (2004) seminal research on the English context is that spiritualism reflected some of the gender politics of the Victorian age. In brief, women's interest in these practices is seen as both a subversion of existing gender power relations and a reflection of their emerging status and autonomy.
4. 'New Age' is a social movement incorporating diverse goals but which are likely to promote a variety of personal and interpersonal values such as self-responsibility, psychological growth and creativity (see English-Lueck 1990:

1). A range of key texts have provided timely analyses into understanding the nature of 'New Age' healing practices in both British and American society (McGuire 1988; Hess 1993; Heelas 1996; Brown 1997; Prince and Riches 2000; McClean 2006).

5. The historical evidence surrounding the use of gemstones and crystals for healing purposes is seemingly scant, and it is not the place to discuss the literature here. However, some healing texts frequently cite the origins of crystal healing in Egypt, where stones such as malachite were said to be used for healing and protection (Raven 2005); origins in Ayurvedic medicine have also been discussed (see Adler and Mukherji 1995; Beckman 1997). Crystal and crystalline structures have been used throughout history as both artefact and metaphor, symbolically representative of transcendence and spiritual transformation, most commonly noted in alchemy and the mythology of the philosopher's stone or *lapis* (Holy Grail) (see Bletter 1981).
6. In the House of Lords (2000) report, crystal healing is placed in the third group or tier of therapies, which 'lack any credible evidence base'. Spiritual healing, somewhat contradictorily, sits in the second group, which act to 'complement conventional medicine'.
7. All names of places and people have been changed to protect the anonymity and confidentiality of the participants in the study.
8. Schneirov and Geczik (2002: 211) also note that these difficult personal experiences led to people developing an interest in alternative medicine. In addition, Warkentin (2000: 214) highlights recovery from cancer as being the personal motivation for one particular healer in Canada.
9. These theories have not been exclusively applied to alternative healers; Löyttyniemi (2005) explores the use of illness stories amongst conventional medical doctors.
10. The word 'sensitive' is used by healers to describe individuals who are perceived as embodying some special abilities, through which they experience more acutely a connection with the spirit world.
11. 'Tumbled': a crystal that is rounded, with no rough or terminated edges.
12. The 'soul star' refers to a chakra point that is extended approximately six inches above the top of the head (Raphaell 1990: 29).

References

Adler, L.L. and B.R. Mukherji (eds). 1995. *Spirit Versus Scalpel: Traditional Healing and Modern Psychotherapy*. Westport, CT: Bergin and Garvey.

Alver, B.G. 1995. 'The Bearing of Folk Belief on Cure and Healing', *Journal of Folklore Research* 32(1): 21–33.

Barrow, L. 1986. *Independent Spirits: Spiritualism and English Plebeians, 1850–1920*. London: Routledge.

Beckman, H. 1997. *Mantras, Yantras and Fabulous Gems: Healing Secrets of the Ancient Vedas*. New Delhi: Balaji Publishing.

Benor, D.J. 1984. 'Psychic Healing', in J.W. Salmon (ed.) *Alternative Medicines: Popular and Policy Perspectives*. London: Tavistock.

Bletter, R.H. 1981. 'The Interpretation of the Glass Dream-Expressionist Architecture and the History of the Crystal Metaphor', *Journal of the Society of Architectural Historians* 40(1): 20–43.

Braude, A. 1989. *Radical Spirits: Spiritualism and Women's Rights in Nineteenth Century America*. Boston, MA: Beacon Press.

Brown, M.F. 1997. *The Channeling Zone: American Spirituality in an Anxious Age*. Cambridge, MA: Harvard University Press.

Easthope, G. 1986. *Healers and Alternative Medicine: A Sociological Examination*. Aldershot: Gower.

Edgar, I.R. 1995. *Dreamwork: Anthropology and the Caring Professions*. Aldershot: Avebury.

English-Lueck, J.A. 1990. *Health in the New Age: A Study in Californian Holistic Practices*. Albuquerque, NM: University of New Mexico Press.

Fadlon, J. 2004. "Meridians, Chakras and Psycho-Neuro-Immunology: The Dematerialising Body and the Domestication of Alternative Medicine', *Body and Society* 10(4): 69–86.

Fisch, S. 1968. 'Botanicas and Spiritualism in a Metropolis', *Milbank Memory Fund Quarterly* 46: 377–88.

Frankenberg, R. 1986. 'Sickness as Cultural Performance: Drama, Trajectory, and Pilgrimage Root Metaphors and the Making Social of Disease', *International Journal of Health Services* 16(4): 603–26.

Frohock, F.M. 1992. *Healing Powers: Alternative Medicine, Spiritual Communities, and the State*. Chicago: University of Chicago Press.

Gerber, R. 2001. *Vibrational Medicine: The Number 1 Handbook of Subtle Energy*. Rochester, VT: Bear and Company.

Glik, D.C. 1988. 'Symbolic, Ritual and Social Dynamics of Spiritual Healing', *Social Science and Medicine* 27(11): 1197–1206.

______. 1990. 'The Redefinition of the Situational Construction of Spiritual Healing Experiences', *Sociology of Health and Illness* 12(2): 151–68.

Heelas, P. 1996. *The New Age Movement: Religion, Culture and Society in the Age of Postmodernity*. Oxford: Blackwell.

Hess, D.J. 1993. *Science in the New Age: The Paranormal, Its Defenders and Bunkers, and American Culture*. Madison: University of Wisconsin Press.

House of Lords. 2000. 'Complementary and Alternative Medicine', report of the Select Committee on Science and Technology, HL Paper 123. London: HMSO.

Hufford, D.J. 1988. 'Contemporary Folk Medicine', in N. Gevitz (ed.) *Other Healers: Unorthodox Medicine in America*. Baltimore, MD: John Hopkins University Press.

Lee, J.A. 1976. 'Social Change and Marginal Therapeutic Systems', in R. Wallis and P. Morley (eds), *Marginal Medicine*. London: Peter Owen.

Löyttyniemi, V. 2005. 'Doctors as Wounded Storytellers: Embodying the Physician and Gendering the Body', *Body and Society* 11(1): 87–110.

McClean, S. 2003. 'Doctoring the Spirit: Exploring the Use and Meaning of Mimicry and Parody at a Healing Centre in the North Of England', *Health* 7(4): 483–500.

——. 2005. "The Illness Is Part of the Person": Discourses of Blame, Individual Responsibility and Individuation at a Centre for Spiritual Healing in the North Of England', *Sociology of Health and Illness* 27(5) 628–648.

——. 2006. *An Ethnography of Crystal and Spiritual Healers in Northern England: Marginal Medicine and Mainstream Concerns*. Lewiston, NY: Edwin Mellen Press.

McGuire, M.B. (with D. Kantor). 1988. *Ritual Healing in Suburban America*. New Brunswick, NJ: Rutgers University Press.

Napolitano, V. and G.M. Flores. 2003. 'Complementary Medicine: Cosmopolitan and Popular Knowledge, and Transcultural Translations: Cases from Urban Mexico', *Theory, Culture and Society* 20(4): 79–95.

O'Connor, B.B. 1995. *Healing Traditions: Alternative Medicine and the Health Professions*. Philadelphia: University of Pennsylvania Press.

——. 2000. 'Conceptions of the Body in Complementary and Alternative Medicine', in M. Kelner and B. Wellman (eds), *Complementary and Alternative Medicine: Challenge and Change*. Amsterdam: Harwood Academic Publishers.

Oppenheim, J. 1985. *The Other World: Spiritualism and Psychical Research in England, 1850–1914*. Cambridge: Cambridge University Press.

Owen, A. 2004. *The Darkened Room: Women, Power and Spiritualism in Late Victorian England*, 2nd edn. Chicago: University of Chicago Press.

Prince, R. and D. Riches. 2000. *The New Age in Glastonbury: The Construction of Religious Movements*. Oxford: Berghahn.

Raphael, K. 1990. *The Crystalline Transmission: A Synthesis of Light*. Sante Fe, NM: Aurora Press.

Raven, H. 2005. *Heal Yourself with Crystals: Crystal Medicine for Body, Emotions and Spirit*. London: Godsfield Press.

Sample, I. 2007. 'Homeopathy Science Degrees "Gobbledygook"', *Guardian*, 2 March.

Schneirov, M. and J.D. Geczik. 2002. 'Alternative Health and the Challenges of Institutionalization', *Health* 6(2): 201–20.

Sharma, U. 1992. *Complementary Medicine Today: Practitioners and Patients*. London: Routledge.

Singh, J. 1992. *The Yoga of Vibration and Divine Pulsation*. Albany, NY: State University of New York Press.

Skultans, V. 1974. *Intimacy and Ritual: A Study of Spiritualism, Mediums and Groups*. London: Routledge and Kegan Paul.

Snow, L.F. 1978. 'Sorcerers, Saints and Charlatans: Black Folk Healers in Urban America', *Culture, Medicine and Psychiatry* 2: 69–106.

Synnott, A. 1992. 'Tomb, Temple, Machine and Self: The Social Construction of the Body', *British Journal of Sociology* 43(1): 79–110.

Warkentin, R. 2000. 'Creative Response to Alternative Medicine: Clients of a Modern Finnish Healer in a Northwestern Ontario City', *Qualitative Health Research* 10(2): 214–24.

WHO. 2002. 'World Health Organization Traditional Medicine Strategy, 2002–2005'. Geneva: WHO.

Chapter 8

Medical Pluralism in the Republic of Ireland: Biomedicines as Ethnomedicines

Anne MacFarlane and Tomas de Brún

Introduction

This chapter is concerned with the relationship between diverse medical systems as they co-exist in the Republic of Ireland over time. We offer an overview of the history of folk medicine in Ireland, as well as analysis of 'alternative' and 'complementary' medicine use and the practice of biomedicine with reference to resistance and allegiances within majority and minority communities.

We draw on research conducted during the 1990s about traditions of folk healing, their relationships with more recent alternative and complementary medicine and the positioning of Western biomedicine as the formal, sanctioned healthcare system. These empirical data are put in dialogue with a more recent study about refugee and asylum seekers' experiences of general practice.[1] Findings about the heterogeneity of refugee and asylum seekers' treatment strategies and the way in which some of these expand the character of plural medicine in Ireland are of interest to us with particular reference to the language(s) of biomedicine(s). We argue that the legitimacy of Western biomedicine as it is practiced in Irish general practice is being questioned by communities from Eastern Europe. In response to this, refugees and asylum seekers use diverse treatment strategies, with the most frequent response being to draw on biomedicine from their 'home' countries. Thus, while studies of medical pluralism typically focus on heterogeneity between different forms of medicine (with biomedicine as the dominant form), these data highlight the enactment of a greater heterogeneity within biomedicine itself. This leads us to the view that within studies of medical pluralism we need to approach biomedicine as a diverse and plural set of culturally mediated practices and sets of discourses.

Medical Pluralism: Mapping the Terrain

Medical pluralism occurs where different medical systems, with different underlying philosophies, co-exist and compete with each other at any given time (Janzen 1978). A longstanding view within biomedicine has been that medical pluralism is about localised, indigenous practices that are inconsistent with, and inferior to, Western biomedicine.

This view can be traced back to the nineteenth century when the scientific foundations of modern Western biomedicine were developed, most specifically with the emergence of the germ-theory doctrine of aetiology and scientific discoveries about links between micro-organisms and certain diseases. These scientific developments meant that, for the first time, the work of biomedicine was deemed superior to that of 'irregular' healers in Western societies and beyond. This laid down the developments of the biomedical model of health which states that all diseases or physical disorders can be explained by disturbances in physiological processes which result from injury, biochemical imbalances, and bacterial or viral infections. The subsequent development of antibiotics to cure illnesses caused by bacterial infection, the availability of state support through legislation and technical changes in the nature of medical practice, were major factors which contributed to and 'sealed' the hegemonic status of biomedicine in the modern period (see Friedson 1975).

The implications of this for other systems of medicine were significant. The broad stereotype within biomedicine was that people across cultures were assumed to lack systematic health beliefs and therapies until Western biomedicine was available. With the 'discovery' of scientific biomedicine, other existing systems were no longer considered worthy of use. The 'task' as it were was to spread biomedicine across Western and non-Western societies and eradicate the need for, or use of, folk healing and spiritual practices.[2]

Clearly, this was an ethnocentric perspective that saw health practices beyond the domain of biomedicine as 'other' and inferior.[3] Anthropologists have always contended ethnocentricity in biomedicine (see Goldstein 2004), giving extensive attention to the plurality of health practices in different settings and, furthermore, the legitimacy of these (e.g., Pillsbury 1978). Over time, anthropologists have contributed to a broadening of perspectives within the biomedical profession by emphasising that different medical systems co-exist with each other in almost all societies and, furthermore, that these persist over time even with the availability of biomedicine. For instance, Lambert (1996) describes how, in Rajasthan, biomedicine has simply contributed to a widening of the range of treatment strategies that are available. Biomedicine has thus not entirely replaced local forms of therapy; nor does use of indigenous treatments indicate resistance to, or rejection of, biomedicine.

More recently, the use of alternative or complementary medicines was taken as a sign of resistance to biomedicine but this has not been borne out either in empirical research in the U.K. (Thomas Carr and Westlake 1991; Sharma 1995; Saks 2006), the U.S.A (Eisenberg et al. 1993), Australia (Lloyd, Lupton and Hasleton 1993), or Canada (Northcott and Bachynsky 1993), where concurrent use of systems is very evident. As with the use of traditional indigenous forms of care and healing in non-Western societies, the use of alternative and complementary therapies in Western societies is best understood as a practice that is closely associated with people's circumstances, knowledge domains within their social networks and the availability of different treatments.

Studies of medical pluralism have paid less attention to health practices of migrant communities in Western societies. Those that have taken this focus offer interesting opportunities to learn about the heterogeneity of health practices across the dichotomy of 'folk' and so-called newer alternative or complementary medicines.[4]

Rao's (2006) study of Asian Indian migrants in the U.S.A. revealed that they have a range of choices available to them, including traditional folk remedies, Ayurveda, homeopathy and allopathy.

Mostly there is a preference to use traditional home remedies based on Ayurvedic principles when ill, with visits to allopathic doctors for more serious illnesses. It is common for people to use traditional systems when at home in India and, also, to bring over-the-counter traditional medicines back to the U.S.A. for treatment of major and minor illnesses. The authors describe a broad pattern of counter acculturation for minor illness and acculturation for major illness as noted in this research.

Similar findings were reported by Green et al. (2006) in their study of Chinese immigrants in the U.K. Women who are more 'connected' with majority English culture are more successful in their consultations with Western healthcare practitioners. At the same time, there is evidence of the dual use of systems, pragmatic responses to illness and a willingness to use whatever therapy is available. Reasons for use of Chinese medicine in the U.K. is, in part, linked to experienced barriers to healthcare, including language barriers and mixed experiences with interpreters; there are examples of errors and misdiagnoses given by the women in their accounts. Their awareness of linguistic and conceptual communication problems means that these women are sometimes reluctant to visit Western doctors.

In this study, over half of the sample report that they sometimes seek Chinese medical treatment from 'home'. Medicines are sent over from home and practitioners are consulted during visits home. There were also many examples of visits being made specifically for medical purposes. One reported benefit of these consultations at 'home' is that it is easier to have meaningful dialogue with a doctor because it is easier to express oneself. The authors rightly point out that this finding perhaps signals an increase in the globalisation of healthcare and offers further opportunities for medical pluralism.

Another study with Chinese women considered that the maintenance of indigenous health beliefs is seen not only as a product of exclusion from Western healthcare but is also related to identity. The use of Chinese medicine demonstrates 'one is still Chinese after all' whereas privileging Western medicine asserts that 'one is "modern"' (Gervais and Jovchelovitch 1998). What emerges from this analysis is that identity is a fluid reality shaping, and being shaped by, treatment strategies and experiences across medical systems.

What this body of research demonstrates is that medical pluralism is universal and omnipresent. The authors of this chapter acknowledge that practitioners and patients alike operate within a socio-cultural context where a plurality of medicines is available and utilized differentially with reference to the social positioning and preferences of the actors in question. This chapter is, therefore, not an attempt to confirm the credentials of medical pluralism. Rather, it takes medical pluralism as a given and a starting point, and seeks instead to broaden our understanding of medical pluralism itself to include biomedicines. In this context, 'biomedicines' refers to the various ways biomedicine is mediated differently through different socio-cultural systems and different socio-cultural expressions of biomedicine.

References to medical pluralism often refer to a heterogeneity of medicines rooted in different ethnic, folk, cultural practices and beliefs, and/or a host of unconventional healing practices (Kaptchuk and Eisenberg 2001) offered through a variety of alternative medicines or complementary medicines. It is noteworthy, for instance, that Kaptchuk and Eisenberg's recent taxonomy of medical pluralism in a major medical journal seems to endorse biomedicine as normative by failing to position it within the taxonomy of medical pluralism (ibid.) This also suggests a view of biomedicine as a unitary system, which it is not.[5]

In this chapter, we present data generated in Ireland through the Communication with Asylum Seekers and Refugees (CARe) project. This project was conducted from the Department of General Practice, National University of Ireland, Galway with Croatian, Serbian, Russian, and Ukrainian members of the refugee and asylum-seeking communities who are living in Galway city on the west coast of Ireland. Our analysis suggests that members of these populations are happy to operate a form of medical pluralism that includes active differentiation of forms of biomedicine and choices between utilising different socio-cultural presentations of biomedicine. If the literature usually presents biomedicine as part of a range of choices between it and other unconventional forms of healing, refugees and asylum seekers in the CARe project predominantly[6] engage in an exercise of choice *between* biomedicines. The data presented from these communities suggests an acceptance, comfort with, and belief in biomedicine as their key (though not exclusive) avenue to healing; yet it also highlights that biomedicine as refugees and asylum seekers have experienced it in an Irish context through interactions with their GPs in Galway is not offering them the service they need or expect.

Our position in this chapter is that refugee and asylum-seeker dissatisfaction is less to do with a simple unmediated mechanics of how GP services are delivered in Galway than it has to do with the mismatch between different socio-cultural presentations of biomedicine offered differentially in Galway, Croatia, Serbia, Russia and the Ukraine. The key theme of this chapter, supported by the evidence, is that medical pluralism can be extended to include biomedicines understood as different socio-cultural mediations of biomedicine. As a practice, biomedicine is mediated differently depending on location and cultural context. This means that biomedicine itself is a socio-cultural product.[7] The fact that biomedicine is science does not make it culture-neutral, or beyond the reach of cultural influence or accretions. In terms of its delivery, biomedicine becomes a recognisably different 'thing' in different places. While the above general point has long been accepted within socio-cultural and medical anthropology and medical sociology, we believe that, within an Irish context at least, the practical implications of the above are insufficiently understood – and, at a broader level, within the wider biomedical literature, it may be insufficiently acknowledged.

The following section offers an overview of medical pluralism in Ireland. We draw on research conducted during the 1990s about traditions of folk healing, their relationships with more recent alternative and complementary medicine and the positioning of Western biomedicine as the formal, sanctioned healthcare system. These empirical data are put in dialogue with the more recent CARe project about refugee and asylum-seekers' experiences of general practice in order to elucidate further relationships with biomedicine in the Irish context and to consider these in relation to plural health practices among majority and minority communities.

Medical Pluralism in Ireland

We know from Ireland's cultural heritage that generations of communities relied on indigenous folk medicines and folk healers. A national scheme, designed by the Folklore Commission of Ireland, produced a wealth of information about socio-cultural health practices of the time. The Schools Scheme 1937–1938, as it was called, invited senior-class pupils in primary schools around the country to record folklore from their parents, grandparents and neighbours as part of their homework. The endeavour represented an attempt to gather details of important local knowledge and practices from older generations because of fears that this information was dying out and in danger of being lost. The complete archive is available at the Department of Irish Folklore, University College Dublin. Some of the issues explored in the Schools Scheme relate to indigenous folk medicines, folk healers and the use of holy wells.

The unique methodology of the 1930s folklore scheme was used as a means of re-examining contemporary health practices in the 1990s (Murphy 1995). The practice and prevalence of traditional folk medicine in Ireland in the 1990s, defined as home cures, herbal remedies, the use of folk healers (including bone-setters and faith healers), knowledge and use of newer alternative and complementary medicines not indigenous to Ireland (defined as acupuncture, reflexology, homoeopathy), and recourse to biomedicine (defined as GP visits and hospital use) were examined.

A total of 133 children's essays were obtained from 11 primary schools in the rural Burren region of County Clare, while another 386 essays were obtained from 10 primary schools in Cork city, the second largest city in the Republic of Ireland. This research was developed further (MacFarlane 1998) with a national interview study of older people's health practices across medical systems from their childhood to the present day. Fifty-one interviews with older people were conducted, all of whom would have been in primary school at the time of the original Schools Scheme. The purpose of the interviews was not to recollect participation in the folklore scheme but to locate socio-cultural health practices of the 1930s in a longer trajectory from participants' childhood through adult life, middle age and their older years.

These studies produced a wealth of knowledge about medical pluralism in Ireland. From content analysis of the children's essays we learned that knowledge of folk medicine was high in the rural Burren area (Murphy and Kelleher 1995) but lower in the urban setting of Cork city. Overall, patterns of use were low in both settings. It was found that people from lower socio-economic groups were more likely to report use of traditional folk remedies while those from higher income groups were more likely to report use of alternative or complementary medicine (MacFarlane and Kelleher 1997). From the survey of children's essays, there was evidence of a strong allegiance to biomedicine with regular GP contact, experience of hospital visits and overall satisfaction with the provision of care.

In-depth analysis of the completed interviews with older people revealed that, as expected, use of folk medicine was commonplace in interviewees' childhoods. Details of herbal remedies and magico-religious cures (Yoder 1972) were recorded. Garlic was considered valuable to prevent colds and flu, and soup made from boiled nettles collected in May was cited as a preventive treatment as well as cleansing blood and promoting good health. Herbs and food items were also used to treat illness: a mixture of boiled milk, onions and pepper was frequently mentioned as a good treatment for colds; slices of raw potato were laid over burns to heal and sooth; and poultices were made to treat festered wounds using bread and boiled water.

Details of folk healers were recorded across both studies. There were references to bone-setters, seventh sons of seventh sons (believed to have healing powers because of their birth order), women who married men with the same surname (for example, if a McCarthy married a McCarthy), and faith healers. The older people were very cautious about complementary medicine. Few had used such medicine and several commented that they would only consider doing so if their GP advised that course of action. This sense of allegiance to biomedicine was very common in older people's accounts.

In recent years, Ireland has quite rapidly become more multicultural due to unprecedented inward migration (MacEinri 2001), which includes the arrival of refugees and asylum seekers. This demographic shift has implications for medical pluralism and its relationship with healthcare provision in Ireland (MacFarlane and Ginnety 2001). In the following section we examine data from a relatively recent study with Croatian, Serbian, Russian and Ukrainian members of the refugee and asylum-seeking communities in Galway city. The aim of the CARe project was to explore the impact of language as a barrier to primary care services for refugees and asylum seekers living in Ireland, with a specific objective being to document people's experiences of accessing and using GP services.

Following recommendations for best practice in research with new ethnic minority communities in Ireland (Feldman, Frese and Yousif 2002), participatory learning and action (PLA) methods (Chambers 1994; O' Reilly-de Brún and de Brún 2003) were used. A major feature of this research has been the use of a peer-researcher model, whereby four Eastern Europeans acted as peer researchers for data collection.

Refugees and asylum seekers who had experience of accessing and using general-practice services in Galway city with little or no English were of interest for the research. Purposeful sampling (Patton 1990), disaggregated by ethnicity (Croatian, Serbian, Ukrainian, Russian) and gender was used. The focus on Serbo-Croat- and Russian-speaking communities was a function of the ethnicity and language skills of the peer-researcher group.[8] Twenty-six participants completed the research, sixteen women and ten men. At the time of data collection, ten were asylum seekers, six had refugee status and ten had residency in Ireland on the basis of having Irish-born children.[9]

The collected data revealed details of heterogeneous treatment strategies to which we will now turn in order to develop our thesis that medical pluralism can be extended to include biomedicines, understood as different socio-cultural mediations of biomedicine.

Biomedicines: Greater Inclusivity in Medical Pluralism

Throughout the CARe study, 'language' was understood to mean the spoken languages of refugees and asylum seekers in the study, given that the language used within GP practices in the Republic of Ireland is English.[10] Participants reported employing a range of personal strategies to overcome the language barrier. These included employing the assistance of informal interpreters in the person of spouses, friends and children, coupled with the use of gestures, body language, the use of dictionaries and phrase books, and memorising phrases. Some unexpected aspects of a number of these strategies proved successful, particularly in the sense of support offered by informal interpreters who were friends or family. Beyond this support, participants said that such interpreters were not necessarily very good at speaking English, and that this did not always assist communication with the GP. It was also clear that using friends and family as interpreters raised issues of confidentiality for patients, and that while people with 'good' English tended to emerge as leaders, they were not always liked or trusted within their small communities. A further important point was that even those participants who had good English emphasised the difficulties they had experienced in their consultations.

Poor Communication and GP Attitudes

After a discussion about pros and cons regarding the use/non-use of formal interpreters within Irish GP services, participants acknowledged the poor quality of communication between themselves and GPs even though they, as patients, expended a great deal of energy in efforts which they hoped would improve communication. The net effect of such poor communication from a refugee and asylum-seeker perspective produced a reflection on GP attitudes. Participants experienced the message conveyed by GPs during consultations as often being one of impatience, anger, indifference and annoyance where the GP seemed to be 'switched off' and not to be listening. There was a view among participants that their lack of language competence was equated with a lack of intelligence by GPs, which they found shocking and offensive. They were suspicious that they were being given prescriptions with the aim, as one person put it, just 'to get rid of us'. Encounters with GPs in general (with some notable exceptions) left refugees and asylum seekers anxious, stressed, feeling nervous before the consultation and exhausted after it.

Questioning GP Competence rather than Biomedicine

It is clear from the CARe data that poor communication and negative GP attitudes and behaviours resulted in an experience for refugees and asylum seekers in the Galway area that, at best, was less than ideal, and constituted an impediment to the healing of illness. According to the data, the response from refugees and asylum seekers to this unhappy situation was to question the competency of the GPs in question. Participants referred to their perceptions of misdiagnoses, the use of incorrect procedures, a lack of clinical competence, and differences in GP style when generating GP narratives.[11]

Participants also acknowledged that while they questioned the competencies of Irish GPs based on their own observations, it was very difficult for them to check out these observations with their GP because of their own poor English-language ability or poor quality translation and interpretation where formal interpreters were available. It wasn't unusual for participants to say that maybe their GP was good but they couldn't verify this because of the language barrier.

The key point we wish to make here is that the research group questioned GP competencies based on their experiences of biomedicine in their home countries. Their knowledge of biomedicine was drawn from their experience of having been patients within the biomedical systems of Croatia, Serbia, Russia and the Ukraine respectively. Much of their critique of GP practice as they experienced it in Ireland was premised on their previous contact and 'formation' as patients routinely exposed to biomedicine as Croats, Serbs, Russians and Ukrainians. Whether the issue of the perceived incompetence of Irish GPs is related to hygiene management, incorrect procedures being used to take blood pressure, the issuing of inappropriate prescriptions, or differences in GP style when generating patient narratives, it is our contention that part of the barrier to communication experienced by both participants, and presumably GPs, was the differing ways that biomedicine is mediated in different socio-cultural contexts. In our view, what is happening in the Galway context is not a rejection of biomedicine, but represents a difficulty refugees and asylum seekers have with biomedicine as it is offered in this particular Irish (or more properly, Galway) socio-cultural manifestation. Also, Galway GPs are judged to be less than adequate not by some set of criteria drawn from other unconventional (ethnic, folk, alternative or complementary) forms of medicine, but by the criteria of biomedicine itself –though these criteria are rooted in the patients' experience of biomedicine in their 'home' countries. Thus, we believe that a case can be made for including in our understanding of medical pluralism a place for foregrounding differing socio-cultural mediations of biomedicine, what we call biomedicines (in the plural).

Embracing Biomedicines: Behaviour Post GP-consultations

Further evidence for participants' desire to access biomedicine was given in their accounts of their actions after having experienced specific and accumulative GP consultations. Their behaviours included changing their GP in an effort to gain access to better care, though this did not always prove successful. Participants also talked about reliance on the use of hospital and A&E departments because they considered that hospital and A&E staff made more of an effort to understand what they were saying in order to decipher what they were presenting with. Participants also explained that they sometimes avoided the GP altogether, and some used self-care strategies: one woman talked about using 'alternative medicine' (herbal treatments), and there were frequent accounts of sending shopping lists 'home' for familiar over-the-counter products from pharmacies. Also, some described symptoms over the phone to a family member in their home country and asked them for advice, or sought advice from a known biomedical doctor or sent over specific medications. Some also travelled home for medical care, though this was only possible for those with recognised refugee status in Ireland.

For example, two participants said they would like to change GP but wondered whether things would be any better. Another participant also had a lot of problems finding a GP she was happy with. She had changed doctors twice and was now with a third GP, who she was happier with. However, it was still very hard to explain things to her GP and she still tended to go straight to A&E. Meanwhile, one respondent said that she felt completely isolated from her GP and the primary care services. She had refugee status at the time and was waiting to go home for treatment. Finally, one participant had a skin condition that she could not explain to doctors in Ireland. She knew the prescription cream she needed and had a prescription in Latin with her (from home) which her Irish GP said he could not understand. Her Irish GP offered her something else but she wanted to use the cream that she has used previously. On other occasions, she phoned home and asked her mother (who works in a hospital) to discuss her case with doctors and see if she could come up with a diagnosis and some advice.

Our analysis indicates that over a third of the sample were accessing either the services of biomedical practitioners in their home country, or accessing products that are generally sanctioned and legitimated by biomedical authorities in the home country. All of the above underlines the acceptance of biomedicine as the favoured form of medicine by refugees and asylum seekers in the Galway area. While we typically think of medical pluralism as offering heterogeneity of different forms of medicine, including where biomedicine is the dominant form, the data from the CARe project would seem to suggest that, as far as those involved in the research are concerned, there is a heterogeneity within biomedicine itself. This again leads us to the view that we need to approach biomedicine as a diverse and plural set of culturally mediated practices and discourses.

From Language Barrier to Languages of Communication

While the explicit focus of the CARe project was on the language barrier, where 'language' is understood to mean 'spoken language competency', the evidence presented above suggests language in this narrow sense (though vitally important in itself, and foundational in our understanding of problems encountered by refugees and asylum seekers in GP consultations in Galway) is only part of a whole repertoire of communication events that occurs within the context of GP consultations. Examining this repertoire of communication events extends our analysis beyond communication exclusively understood as a spoken language event to include a consideration of other languages of communication utilised by refugees and asylum seekers. These other languages of communication are drawn from that reservoir commonly referred to as 'culture'. These are far less obvious, more subtle and intangible than spoken language, but nonetheless constitute a crucially important content in terms of the tone of the encounter, displays and readings (and misreadings) of body language, differing (patient and practitioner) expectations in terms of consultation style and delivery, and even different understandings and ways of approaching how the body can be described, or should be accessed in terms of the medical examination itself.

Though 'culture' is about differing contents, at another level it is also about processes. This is particularly so when individuals and groups employ different forms of 'cultural capital' (Bourdieu 1986) in the assertion of issues related to identity maintenance and/or identity assertion. When this happens, individuals and groups deploy culture as a political tool. Utilising culture in this way is often a strategy used in cross-cultural encounters and exchanges, particularly where the actors involved occupy different positions vis-à-vis their access to social power and status. The deployment of cultural capital can be a powerful tool in asserting individual or group identity or challenging dominant power configurations.

In Ireland, refugees and asylum seekers occupy a relatively powerless position and the GP consultation may be for them a particularly painful moment of being reminded of this. It would be surprising if they failed to employ some cultural capital in the form of asserting the superiority of Eastern European biomedicines as a way of asserting an identity and agency within an otherwise very alienating and disempowering situation and context.

Conclusion: Biomedicines as Ethnomedicines

In this chapter, we have shown that traditions of Irish indigenous folk medicine remain, certainly in terms of people having knowledge of remedies and practices. Newer alternative and complementary therapies are also available and used. These systems co-exist with the dominant biomedicine, or rather biomedicines in the plural, including Irish biomedicine and other biomedicines. The range of treatment strategies in Ireland has extended. Recourse to medicines from 'home' by refugees and asylum seekers from Eastern European countries has not replaced the use of biomedicine as practised in Galway but is part of a negotiated set of practices within their health-seeking behaviour.

Our findings resonate with other studies which illustrate that dissatisfaction with biomedicine sometimes motivates people to use different treatment strategies. They also resonate with those of Rao (2006) and Green et al. (2006), in that migrant communities seek medicines from their 'home' countries. What is unusual or additional in the present case, however, is that these refugees and asylum seekers were not necessarily looking for an alternative form of medicine from home, but for familiar biomedicine. We acknowledge that the socio-economic status of participants is likely to be relevant here. Under the Irish General Medical Scheme, refugees and asylum seekers are entitled to a medical card, which provides them with free GP and hospital care. Fees for alternative and complementary therapies, however, are not covered by medical cards. The allowances for asylum seekers are very low (€19.10 per adult and €9.60 direct provision allowance per child at the time of writing) and would prohibit payment of such fees. However, we do not know how the costs of accessing medicines from home are met and arguably these too put some demand on people's meagre allowances. It would be interesting to learn more about the relationship between their plurality of health practices and socio-economic conditions. For now, however, these data indicate that the movement of the refugees and asylum seekers involved in the project across cultural contexts and 'presentations' of biomedical practice has led to a questioning of the legitimacy of Irish general practice when compared with Eastern European healthcare, and, additionally, an assertion of identity in a context where their ethnic identity is under stress.

This would suggest that the biomedicine available in Ireland is itself an ethnomedicine, just as the biomedicine available in Croatia, Serbia, Russia and the Ukraine is. Biomedicine as ethnomedicine is something Helman talks about, and he reminds us that dominant systems in any society should not be studied in isolation. They do not exist in a social or cultural vacuum; instead they are:

> an expression of and, to some extent a miniature model of, the values and social structures of the society from which it arises. Different types of society therefore produce different types of medical systems and different attitudes to health and illness, depending on their dominant ideology – whether this is capitalist, welfare state, socialist or communist. (Helman 2007: 96)

We would note that the above designations are macro categories, which may account for some of the differences our participants raised between the practice of medicine in Ireland and their home countries. Biomedicines, as we are speaking of them here, are enacted differently in capitalist societies (and by extension any other types of society with their own unique forms of biomedicine). But again, even within capitalist countries and regions within those countries it is our view that variations among biomedicines occur. This highlights the appropriateness of researching biomedicines in the future at a more micro, local level. To this end, in approaching an analysis and understanding of biomedicines at the micro level, ethnographic and participatory-style research may be particularly suited to that task.

In addition, we wish to point to the significance of our presentation of biomedicines as ethnomedicines for the ongoing theoretical consideration of medical pluralism. Along with complementary, alternative and folk medicines, we have demonstrated that biomedicines also represent different socio-cultural enactments within a plural understanding of medicine. This approach acknowledges that all medical/healing systems, including biomedicine, mediate different socio-cultural symbologies, discourses and practices, and should therefore be approached relationally, rather than in isolation. Theoretical understanding and exploration of medical pluralism requires that we investigate not only ethnomedicines but also the relational spaces between ethnomedicines. Such investigations of interstices may also illuminate some of the ways in which culture, as both content and process, is continually (re)generated in the 'contact zones' (Merry 1998) between ethnomedicines, including biomedicines as they have been presented in this chapter.

Notes

1. The research on which this chapter is based was carried out as part of the Communication with Asylum Seekers and Refugees (CARe) Project, a result of funding for Anne MacFarlane from the Irish Health Research Board Health Services Research Fellowship Scheme, 2002–2005.
2. The spread of biomedicine cannot be separated from the colonial endeavour, where the 'white man's burden' was an integral part of that endeavour. This so-called burden involved education, enlightenment through Western value systems, science and religion, and a 'raising up' out of ignorance of what the colonial powers believed to be lower, inferior peoples (see, e.g., Airhihenbuwa 1994; Loomba 1998).
3. Press (1980) argues this with excellent clarity. He gives an overview of definitional classifications of medical systems that have prioritised Western

biomedicine as 'the' medical system whose scientific character renders it superior to 'lay', 'primitive' medicine, and 'magico-religious' healing.

4. In the sense that complementary medicine today is a descendant of traditional and folk medical systems from various parts of the world: 'herbalism from shamanism and folk remedies, chiropractice and osteopathy from bone setting, homoeopathy from early like-cures-like principles, naturopathy from the Hippocratic lineage' (Fulder 1986: 247).
5. Pillsbury writes that 'each culture has produced over the centuries its own adaptive methodologies for coping with illness. These embody an indigenous etiology; that is, a system explaining the occurrence of illness and disease based on the worldview and religious beliefs of the particular people in question. Following from this, biomedicine, like all systems of medicine, is an indigenous etiology' (Pillsbury 1978: 46).
6. In previous informal research with representatives from Nigerian, Ghanaian and Kenyan refugee and asylum-seeker populations in Galway, one of the authors (de Brún) noted evidence emerging for pluralistic practices that included both utilising diagnoses and cures from biomedical practitioners located in the home country, and also from traditional healers and doctors from a person's own ethnic group.
7. From an anthropological and sociological perspective, it is understood that biomedicine is a distinct socio-cultural 'product' in the sense that it arose and developed out of a particular set of historical influences and along a particular historical trajectory to become what it is today. It is thus a product of those histories, rooted in particular places and times, and carries the cultural hallmarks of its origin and development within it even as it has become a universalising discourse, and a set of practices globally. 'Product' is also used here in a weak sense: 'culture' is understood (following Cohen 1997) as that which aggregates peoples and processes, not something *sui generis* or that which exercises a deterministic power over people. 'Culture' is viewed as processual, open-ended, dynamic and fluid, not an 'it' as is the more popular understanding.
8. We know from the peer researchers that these categories of ethnicity are broad ones that do not fully capture the complexity of self-defined ethnicity. For instance, the Croatian peer researcher explained that she was from a Serbian ethnic-minority community living in Croatia, as were many of her participants, or they were in Serb/Croat mixed marriages, which is why they had come to seek asylum in Ireland during, or after, the Bosnian conflict. Related to this, she explained that Serbo-Croat was the language of former Yugoslavia. When countries separated, separate languages were encouraged – Serbian and Croatian. In practice, many continued speaking Serbo-Croat, which was the shared language of our Croatian peer researcher and her participants during data collection.

9. Irish Justice Minister Michael McDowell established a one-off scheme in order to deal with the legal position of foreign parents of Irish-born children who were born before 1 January 2005. Children of foreign nationals born prior to this date automatically received Irish citizenship. The situation changed after the Citizenship Referendum of 2004, which became law on 1 January 1 2005. See: http://www.ireland.com/focus/referendum2004/guide.html for an overview of the issues in this Referendum.
10. The use of English is normative within GP practice in the Republic of Ireland, though in Irish-speaking or Gealtacht areas – which represent a minority of the total population and are largely bilingual – Irish is also used as a medium of communication.
11. The communication style of Irish general practitioners described by participants in this study is consistent with a consultative style as per the Calgary-Cambridge Guide (Silverman, Kurtz and Draper 2005). This style, which emphasises patients' perspectives on their health and illness, fuelled a sense of uncertainty among participants. It made them question whether their general practitioner knew what they were doing. Being asked by their general practitioner 'What do you think it is?' and "Is that (treatment) okay with you?' led them in turn to ask 'Doesn't this GP know what's going on?' and 'How do I know what is wrong?' The peer researchers explained that the consultation style used by doctors in their home countries is much more authoritarian. Patients would not be asked for their opinion or would not question what doctors said. For similar findings, see Brod and Heurtin-Robert's (1992) paper on older Russian émigrés' experiences of consultation styles in the United States.

References

Airhihenbuwa, C.O. 1994. *Health and Culture: Beyond the Western Paradigm*. Thousand Oaks, CA: Sage.

Bourdieu, P. 1986. *Distinction*, trans. R. Nice. London: Routledge And Kegan Paul.

Brod, M. and S. Heurtin-Roberts. 1992. 'Cross Cultural Medicine: A Decade Later. Older Russian Emigres and Medical Care', *Western Journal Of Medicine* 157(3): 333–36.

Chambers, R. 1994. 'The Origins and Practice of Participatory Rural Appraisal', *World Development* 22: 953–69.

Cohen. A. 1997. 'Culture As Identity: An Anthropologists View'. Retrieved 28 February 2008 from: http://Wsrv.Clas.Virginia.Edu/~Tsawyer/DRBR/Cohen.Txt

Eisenberg, D.M., R.C. Kessler, C. Foster, F. Norlock, D.R. Calkins and T.L. Delbanco. 1993. 'Unconventional Medicine in the United States', *New England Journal of Medicine* 328: 246–52.

Feldman, A., C. Frese and T. Yousif. 2002. 'Research Development and Critical Interculturalism: A Study on the Participation of Refugees and Asylum Seekers in Research and Development-based Initiatives', Dublin: Social Science Research Centre, University College Dublin.

Friedson, E. 1975. *Profession of Medicine: A Study of the Sociology of Applied Knowledge*. New York: Dodd, Mead.

Fulder, S. 1986. 'A New Interest In Complementary (Alternative) Medicine: Towards Pluralism in Medicine', *Impact of Science on Society* 36: 235–42.

Gervais, M.C. and S. Jovchelovitch. 1998. 'Health and Identity: The Case of the Chinese Community in England, *Social Science Information* 37: 709–29.

Goldstein, M.S. 2004. 'The Persistence and Resurgence of Medical Pluralism', *Journal of Health Politics Policy and Law* 29(4/5): 925–45.

Green, G., H. Bradby, A. Chan and M. Lee. 2006. '"We Are Not Completely Westernised": Dual Medical Systems and Pathways to Health Care among Chinese Migrant Women in England', *Social Science and Medicine* 62(6): 1498–1509.

Helman, C.G. 2007. *Culture, Health And Illness*, 5th edn. London: Hodder Arnold.

Janzen, J.M. 1978. *The Quest for Therapy in Lower Zaire*. Berkeley: University Of California Press.

Kaptchuk, T.J. and D.M. Eisenberg. 2001. 'Varieties Of Healing, 2: A Taxonomy Of Unconventional Healing Practices', *Annals of Internal Medicine* 135(3): 196–204.

Lambert, H. 1996. 'Popular Therapeutics and Medical Preferences in Rural North India', *The Lancet* 348: 1706–9.

Lloyd, P., D. Lupton and S. Hasleton. 1993. 'Choosing Alternative Therapy: An Exploratory Study of Sociodemographic Characteristics and Motives of Patients Resident in Sydney', *Australian Journal of Public Health* 17: 135–45.

Loomba, A. 1998. *Colonialism/Postcolonialism*. London: Routledge.

MacEinri, P. 2001. 'Immigration Into Ireland: Trends, Policy Responses, Outlook'. Cork: Irish Centre For Migration Studies, University College Cork.

MacFarlane, A. 1998. 'Medical Pluralism In Ireland 1930s–1990s', unpublished Ph.D. thesis. Galway: National University Of Ireland.

MacFarlane, A. and P. Ginnety. 2001. 'Boiled Nettles in May: Studies of Plural Medicine in Northern and Southern Ireland', in M. Maclachlan (ed.)

Cultivating Health: Cultural Perspectives On Promoting Health. Chichester: Wiley.

MacFarlane, A. and C. Kelleher. 1997. 'Contemporary Health Practices in Ireland: Manual versus Non-manual Differences', *Irish Medical Journal* 90: 240.

Merry, S.E. 1998. 'Law, Culture and Cultural Appropriation', *Yale Journal of Law and the Humanities* 10: 101–29.

Murphy, A. 1995. 'Contemporary Health Practices In Ireland: An Urban–Rural Analysis', unpublished Masters' thesis. Galway: National University Of Ireland.

Murphy, A. and C. Kelleher. 1995. 'Contemporary Health Practices in the Burren, Co Clare', *Irish Journal Of Psychology* 16: 38–51.

Northcott, H.C. and J.A. Bachynsky. 1993. 'Concurrent Utilisation of Chiropractic, Prescription Medicines, Non-prescription Medicines and Alternative Health Care', *Social Science and Medicine* 37: 431–35.

O'Reilly-de Brún, M. and de Brún, T. 2003. 'Participatory Learning and Action Strategies Workshop Manual'. Galway: Centre For Participatory Strategies,.

Patton, M. 1990. *Qualitative Evaluation and Research Methods.* London: Sage.

Pillsbury, B.L.K. 1978. *Traditional Health Care In The Near East.* Washington, DC: United States Agency For International Development.

Press, I. 1980. 'Problems in the Definitions and Classifications of Medical Systems', *Social Science and Medicine* 14B: 45–57.

Rao, D. 2006. 'Choice of Medicine and Hierarchy of Resort to Different Health Alternatives among Asian Indian Migrants in a Metropolitan City in the USA', *Ethnicity and Health* 11(2): 153–67.

Saks, M. 2006. 'The Alternatives To Medicine', in D. Kelleher, J. Gabe and G. Williams (eds), *Challenging Medicine.* London: Routledge.

Sharma, U. 1995. *Complementary Medicine Today: Practitioners And Patients.* London: Routledge.

Silverman, J., S. Kurtz and J. Draper. 2005. *Skills For Communicating with Patients.* Oxford: Radcliffe.

Thomas, K., J. Carr and B. Westlake. 1991. 'Use of Non-Orthodox and Conventional Health Care in Great Britain', *British Medical Journal* 302: 207–10.

Yoder, D. 1972. 'Folk Medicine', in R.Dorson (ed.) *Folklore and Folklife.* Chicago: University Of Chicago Press.

Chapter 9

Born To It and Then Pushed Out of It: Folk Healing in the New Complementary and Alternative Medicine Marketplace

Geraldine Lee-Treweek

Introduction

Folk healers face considerable challenges in the British marketplace of healing. In many ways they could be said to be the poor cousins of other healers who have come to be known as complementary and alternative medicine (CAM) practitioners and many of whom are increasingly recognised by a range of professional groups and society at large. Folk healers, however, remain in the shadows of communities and yet, if we are to believe their accounts, fulfil important health and well-being roles for some people.

These marginalised healers do not have the market position of their CAM counterparts. Often shunning certificated training courses they more often than not see their skills as a birthright, or at least endowed through early experiences that 'naturally' developed their healing abilities. It is this position that completely goes against current thinking about non-medically trained individuals working in health and well-being capacities. There is an increasingly accepted assumption within U.K. society that individuals cannot do (or perhaps should not do) anything with or to anyone else without training and qualifications, and many groups working in health and social care also have to 'prove' their skills. A pertinent example is the way bathing and washing have become certificated activities of caring. There are specialist courses in bathing older people or helping people with learning disabilities to wash and so forth (see, e.g., Twigg 2000, 2003). In the same way, healing – a set of skills once believed to be inherent in the community and usually dispensed through the knowledge and experience of women (Chamberlain 1981) – has now been organised into separate modalities with boundaries and systems of knowledge distribution. It would be wrong to suggest, however, that all CAMs are at such an organised stage, though most show signs of moving towards this. It also cannot be ignored that aspects of CAM have become the province of entrepreneurs of healing, such as those who claim to pass on the skills of healing for a fee (as in Reiki healing, taught by masters to novices) or individuals who sell certificated courses that claim to provide access to angels (who will both support you as you set up in business as a healer and then aid you with the healing itself – a kind of healing double whammy). CAM skills are big business and, as I have noted elsewhere, cynics might say that training in healing often shares features with pyramid selling, whereby sets of skills are taught to one person who then goes onto teach others (Lee-Treweek and Thomson 2005). In the new marketplace of healing, in which it is CAM that is gaining most ground with public and professional groups alike, folk healers find their claims defined as less legitimate; they are the outsiders whose claims to natural healing skills are not authenticated and so, for many consumers of healing, are less credible.

This chapter examines data from qualitative in-depth interviews with four women who feel that the professionalisation of healing has begun to push them out of the healing marketplace. They all argue that their role and place as traditional folk healers has been undermined by CAM developments towards accreditation, training, continuing professional development and membership of professional bodies. All these women feel that they are 'born' to healing, and feel that their personal justifications for doing healing work are embedded in a sense of ascribed ability, identity, community, family and social relationships. Rejection as healers for these women is, therefore, far more profound than rejection from a hobby or leisure pursuit because all four women see being a healer as a central form of status, linked to their birthright, biography and identity. The chapter explores these women's accounts of what they do and, in particular, their market position in relation to other types of healers. Whilst their accounts indicate that initially they were 'born' to healing, increasingly they see themselves as occupying a position in which their refusal to train others seems to be an act of resistance to what they see as inauthentic healing forms that lack credibility. However, the pressure to train and 'prove' one's healing skills is intense, and, for some of the folk healers, undertaking training was a cynical action that they were considering or had considered to ensure they could continue healing and working with people. The chapter then goes on to discuss what the future might hold for folk healers in a competitive and hostile healing entrepreneurial environment.

A Very Brief History of Healing in Britain

It could be argued that there is a much narrower literature about folk healers than other forms of healer. As Saks (1996) has noted, before the formation of a professionalised and integrated medical profession (mainly through the Medical Registration Act of 1858), there was a diverse field of people who claimed to be able to heal others. Within this open market, lay people competed with physicians, surgeons and apothecaries and yet, if accounts such as Mary Chamberlain's (1981) are to be believed, it is folk healers who provided the mainstay of health knowledge and skills to ordinary people in Britain in the pre-industrial era. Chamberlain argues that folk healing prior to the rise of biomedicine encapsulated a number of healing skills, including the use of prayer and religious incantations, herbal lore and expertise in the making of herbal potions and mineral-based remedies, midwifery skills, use of amulets and charms, basic nursing care and support and knowledge of some common ailments and how to help those with them. It is highly likely that 'wise women' and their male counterparts 'cunning men' (who Chamberlain argues were fewer in number) had more knowledge and skills at their disposal than university-trained physicians and other healers. These folk healers were able to respond to community illness with the benefit of experience-based care and theirs was most probably the main form of expertise available to the ordinary person suffering ailments and afflictions. At the same time, lay care in the home was important, with women being 'typically regarded as capable of dealing with everything from domestic medicine, fractures and burns to infections and surgery' (Saks 2004: 64). However, by the eighteenth century, so-called 'wise women', 'cunning men' and women lay healers in the home were increasingly challenged by the Church, which regarded much healing work as witchcraft (see Chapter 2, this volume, on the historical links between healing and witchcraft).

It was not only the Church that challenged folk and other healers. The 1858 Medical Registration Act began a process of exclusion in which folk healers were faced with a concerted attempt by the newly emerging profession of medicine to construct them as untrustworthy and dangerous charlatans. By the first half of the nineteenth century, the pluralistic healthcare marketplace, which had allowed folk healers a role in healing alongside physicians and others, had diminished. At the same time, the power of orthodox medicine had grown and the discrediting of non-medical healers was an accepted way of dealing with competition (Nicholls 1988). Organised, self-regulated and backed by state support, the newly formed medical profession was able to counter competition and gain a key market advantage. As Bakx (1991) famously notes, other healers found themselves 'eclipsed' by the power and development of biomedical dominance. At this time, folk medicine included any healing practice not undertaken by medicine. The concept was only born much later and in direct opposition to the power of biomedicine. Healing work in the early days of biomedicine can be seen as a group of non-medically trained individuals who made up an undifferentiated mass in terms of power and status. Folk healers and CAM healers were thus working in the same marketplace and many individuals, practising with titles we know today as organised CAM groups had more in common with a folk model of healing than the structured professional activities and identities seen today. For instance, in Yorkshire before the Second World War there was a very well-known practitioner who called himself an osteopath – he was self-taught and used a host of methods that would not be recognised by the osteopathic profession today. Extremely popular, he was visited by large groups of people who arrived in buses at his treatment rooms and would wait in line for 'treatment' for back pain. The treatment was invariably the same; the patient would be hit on the back with a toffee hammer and given a bottle of coloured water (medicine) to take home with them. This character was reportedly highly popular, and had many return customers.[1]

Usually, sociological and historical accounts of the rise of complementary and alternative medicine present the re-emergence and growth in popularity of folk healers in 1960s Britain as a triumph, a time of when 'folk medicine' was rebranded as 'complementary and alternative medicine'. However, the assumption that CAM, as a term or as a movement, embraces folk healers today is unfounded (Wing 1998). As we can see from the following quote from Cecil Helman though, there is confusion, even amongst eminent writers, about whether folk healing is part of CAM or CAM is part of folk healing:

> In the UK, as in other Western societies, this sector [the folk sector] is relatively small and ill defined. While local faith healers, gypsy fortune tellers, clairvoyants, psychic consultants, herbalists and 'wise women' still exist in many rural areas, the forms of diagnosis and healing characteristic of the folk sector are more likely to be found in urban areas, especially in alternative or complementary medicine. (Helman 2006: 107)

In his discussion of the folk sector, Helman includes together diverse groups that one could also categorise as CAM healers, or occultists or New Agers. Using folk healing as a kind of sociological dustbin category, Helman fails to recognise the vast differences between these groups and in doing so he illustrates a fundamental flaw in taxonomy that is common in social science and medical discussion of these matters. Since the mid 1990s there has been a range of developments that have altered how CAM is organised and that has created divisions within 'other' non-orthodox forms of healing. Whilst there is overlap between CAM and folk practitioners, in a taxonomy of healing practices one would most suitably place contemporary folk healing in the U.K. separately from most practices of CAM, many of which are now formalised, codified and bound up with training and structured ideologies of healing.

Increasingly there has been greater focus within CAM upon justifying one's position in the healing marketplace through forming a professional community (Cant and Sharma 1998: 247), enforcing qualification to allow entry into this community, excluding others who are not trained in the same way as oneself, and in so doing protecting the boundaries of one's modality and identity with consumers. Indeed, consumers of CAM expect more from those who treat them today and, within a crowded market place, practitioners contend for custom and market position. Lastly, there is a great deal of time being spent by particular groups in trying to gain social recognition of the scope of expertise of their particular specialism. At the same time as some individuals and groups are following professional projects that they believe will make them distinctive in the CAM business, there are still folk healers who again find themselves on the very fringes of healing, though this time they find themselves on the outskirts of both CAM and orthodox biomedical approaches to health and healing.

Folk healers are just as excluded within CAM as they are in relation to biomedicine, but in different ways. For instance, whilst practising healing is open to all in the U.K., it is very difficult to gain insurance to practice any modality without the sanction of a formally recognised CAM professional body membership or training.[2] As folk healers often see themselves as authentic because, firstly, they are not trained in this manner (they are either 'natural' healers or have been trained through charismatic traditions), and secondly, because they are not part of occupational and professional groups, they can find themselves unable to access public liability and other forms of insurance. Excluded both from the means to make money and the means to gain status as healers, it is perhaps unsurprising that folk healers are easily tempted towards training in CAM to accredit what they see as skills they already have. Of course, most folk healers maintain that money is not a deciding factor in what they do and, indeed, much work gets undertaken for free, for 'pocket money', with a system of barter, and for seemingly altruistic reasons. It is interesting that authors, such as May (1997), suggest that payment is an important requirement within healing settings to stabilise relationships and, in particular, to ensure quality and continuity. For May, altruism and being caring are not suitable motivators to create lasting therapeutic relationships within CAM. From this perspective, folk healers are an outmoded and unpredictable approach to healing.

This chapter argues that whilst folk healing can be seen as an amalgamation of many healing forms and skills (often borrowing from a diverse range of cultural sources and modifying traditional types of healing lore to suit contemporary situations), this group of healers is today under threat of extinction. Essentially, what folk healers can offer no longer suits a consumerist model of health and well-being services in which choice is tempered with public notions of professionalism, qualification and professional identity. Whilst

Bakx's (1991) term 'eclipse' described the temporary obscuring of folk healers from the development of modern scientific medicine up to the mid twentieth century, the situation today may be far more serious for the continuation of the folk healer. As many of the folk healer's skills are swallowed up by more organised CAMs, folk healers now face a crisis of identity, public image and recognition.

Impetus and Methods

This chapter emerges from research with dedicated folk healers working in Staffordshire in the U.K. These are women who are well known and trusted in their localities and who embody an older tradition of community healing often hidden from view from conventional health services. These are quite hard people to find and engage in research because they do not group together or organise themselves in ways that make them traceable; one could say they are mavericks, working as individuals and engaging more with their own local communities than each other.

But these women are not the only impetus for this chapter as in some ways it is a continuation of work I undertook in the past with a character that the four healers would probably wish to distance themselves from – a self-confessed fraudulent healer (Lee-Treweek and Thomson 2005). It is pertinent to spend some time here to consider the features of this fraudster in relation to the notion of the genuine folk healer because by doing this we can more clearly see the public-image problem that modern folk healers face. The idea of a fake healer is a difficult concept because there are many commentators who would regard all notions of healing as fraudulent at worst, and incorrect and misinformed at best. In 2005 I co-authored a paper on the work of Accora, a self-confessed fraudulent healer who was skilled in using the symbols and status of folk healing to make a living.[3] Oddly, she provides an interesting starting point for this discussion as she used her lack of qualifications as a positive way of indicating to those around that she was the 'real deal'. That said, the chance meeting that led to my getting to know Accora was based upon her attending classes to accredit herself in CAM therapies. Whilst Accora had been able to make a good living as a fake folk healer for much of her life, early in 2001 she began to recognise that even she might need at least some certificates on her wall to symbolise her credibility and justify herself to clients.

Accora created a persona of healing based on quite stereotypical notions of what a healer should be, relating to their background, lifestyle, beliefs and powers. Although she lived in a wealthy area of Birmingham, each day Accora made her way to a caravan (that she claimed that she lived in) to await her clientele, surrounded by dream catchers, crystals and tarot cards. Part of Accora's guise was her self-constructed story of Romany heritage and ancestry, although in Accora's more truthful moments she recognised that this was a bastardisation of the reality of her Irish parenthood. Whilst trade had been brisk in the past, she complained that recently she had taken to regularly attending the local spiritualist churches to drum up custom. It was no longer the case that Accora was the only healer around, and people expected more than just symbols, glitter and a good story – they now wanted papers and certificates. At the time of writing the paper about Accora I was fascinated about how this woman made what she claimed to be a good living whilst knowing that the account she gave to people was false. My focus on her was the psychology of the fraudulent psychic rather than Accora's market position or the ways that the professionalisation of healing was affecting her income and personal occupational strategies. That said omitting these factors in my account was a mistake because clearly the heightening need to gain qualifications in healing had forced this fraudster into reconsidering her attitude to costly training. Despite succumbing to the necessity of taking courses, Accora remained sceptical about the quality and nature of the skills she could gain, stating to a colleague of mine that she saw aromatherapy as 'another scam' that she could add to her portfolio. Accora stands as the antithesis to the women discussed in this chapter. The participants discussed here feel that their lives revolve around healing identities that they believe in and feel to be a key part of their identities. However, the folk healers report an increasing struggle to maintain their traditional ways of working in the face of market change towards qualifications and courses.

I began my study after a chance meeting with a woman living in north Staffordshire in 2005. Margaret described herself as a 'healer'. Intrigued to find out more about the type of healing she was involved in, I arranged a meeting and on that first visit was able to carry out initial negotiations with Margaret about carrying out a life-history interview about her work. With great excitement I fairly quickly realised that Margaret was not another CAM therapist but someone whose skills she claimed to have inherited and who was a folk healer. During this first meeting she also used the phrase, 'I was born to it and now I'm just pushed out of it'. This caused me to think about the changing social and market position of healers who have found their skills to be in competition with newer occupational identities and qualifications arising from within CAM. Whilst my study of healing had often focused in the past on CAM practitioners, in particular osteopaths, my interest now turned to how folk healers understood, resisted and accounted for the rise of CAM practitioners, and how this impacted upon their healing work and identities. Using a snowballing technique – making my interests known by word of mouth in health food, crystal and alternative lifestyle shops – I was able to recruit four women who defined themselves as healers and who all lived in the Staffordshire area. All but one person who responded was female. It was quite hard at this stage because many CAM practitioners also responded to my enquiries and I had to decline those who did not fit my categorisation of folk healers. In the end I settled on the following self-made definition:

> Folk healing may be understood to be lay healing that is not carried out under the auspices of formal or recognised CAM modalities but which mobilises a range of healing forms by a non-officially trained practitioner offering services to their local community. Folk healing may therefore be defined not by what healing activities the practitioner actually does but the fact that the practitioner has not been trained through conventionally accepted CAM or other methods.

Working outside formal structures, folk healers can come in many forms and work in a variety of ways. Whilst payment can be part of folk healing, more often than not folk healers mix and match paid healing work with unpaid healing and other forms of paid labour.

I carried out two in-depth interviews with each woman: the first discussing her general life history and experiences, and the second specifically covering social changes around CAM work and the effect of this upon folk healing. These interviews were recorded and analysed thematically. The quotes and information used here in this chapter are from these interviews.

Backgrounds and Beginnings: How Did the Participants Become Healers?

The issue of how and why someone becomes a healer is very important because for the folk healers I interviewed such details operated in lieu of more formal qualifications. All the participants alleged that they had a 'natural' link to healing through birth and/or heritage (that is, heredity). To begin with it is perhaps useful to sketch out some biographical aspects of each folk healer and provide some basic information about them.

Margaret

Margaret was 56, married, and a mother of two grown up children. She had been a healer for as long as she could remember and felt that she was 'born to it'. Margaret reported that her mother had been a healer within her local community, as had her grandmother. Healing was just 'in the blood' and something that the women had just done for others because they demonstrated some natural ability. Margaret reported that her grandmother was involved with a number of other caring duties within the community, including the laying out of dead bodies. Closeness with death, illness and the body were doubtless involved in the development of the personal expertise that contributed to the development of her stock of folk knowledge and which was in turn passed down through the family. Margaret was a part-time administrator for a local government office but only worked as a healer when requested by people she knew or who came to her by word of mouth.

Alex

Alex was 32 and said that she came from Romany traveller heritage. Her background, she felt, had been unconventional, with a family that practised a host of healing and psychic activities, and Alex believed that she had been left with not only healing abilities but also other skills such as clairvoyance and telepathy. Alex put her healing and other attributes down to being around others who were 'gifted' during her childhood and adolescence. She did not believe that she was necessarily born with such skills but she believed the social environment had led to her gaining them from a very early age through being 'in the soup of that stuff'. Whilst she had had a short period in which she began training in spiritual healing, Alex found this formalised setting constraining to her notions of what healing involved and she left after only four months of training to continue healing in her own way. Alex was single and worked in an insurance call centre as a call operative.

Liz

Liz was a forty-year-old homemaker who was married with children, and she saw herself as a 'healer in the true sense', which she argued meant that she had always healed. She even gave examples during the interviews of healing friends as a schoolgirl and knowing that she was 'special in the healing of people and animals'. A housewife with chronically poor health herself (she was badly asthmatic and was troubled with arthritis in her hands and arms), Liz's life seemed full of dealing with other people's problems and worries, and she admitted that this was, at least in part, to take her mind off her own issues. At points in her life Liz had been in receipt of state benefits for ill health and, at the time of the interviews, was looking for a part-time job that would not cause her too many problems with her ongoing illness. Like many healers, though, Liz saw her own suffering as part of a journey into understanding the suffering of others and being able to heal in a deeper way. Liz was also involved with a number of neo-pagan groups that she felt she had affinity with; healing for her was one aspect of an alternative lifestyle.

Maria

Of Italian-migrant heritage, Maria (42) reported being taught the use of herbs, oils, culinary and household products to aid health and healing. Her mother had also used what she termed 'country magic' (such as spells and candle-burning occult activities) to increase the efficacy of remedies but, interestingly, religious prayer also featured in the range of her healing activities. Maria remembered the kitchen as the main space used for healing, with local women from the Italian community coming to their home to have a sitting with her mother. Many other migrant groups had also tended to visit her mother, despite not being of the same cultural heritage, suggesting the possibility of a crossover of folk healing cultures within migrant populations. Maria, who was a teaching assistant, still took her folk healing seriously and, like her mother had done, waited for people to come to her door for help. These days, Maria noted, it was no longer specific ethnic groups she undertook healing work with but anyone who came to know about her skills by word of mouth. Whilst she had continued using a range of folk methods with her own family, she reported mainly concentrating on spiritual healing and spiritual advice to other people. Maria argued that she had suffered from musculoskeletal pain for some time but that her own doctor was at a loss as to why this was. Blood tests and consultant visits had not proved to helpful and Maria believed that her illness may have been due to stress and worry.

Analysis

The biographies of these healers demonstrate a number of similarities. First, they all claimed to have either been born with healing skills or gained them early in childhood through contact with other healers (in all cases these were kin). The role of women in the process of either teaching or encouraging healing skills can clearly be seen, as mothers and grandmothers (but not male family members) are mentioned. All of the participants also shared a sense of wanting more out of life and expressed that healing gave them this. For instance, Liz noted, 'Healing is a very special part of my life … don't get me wrong, motherhood is great and other aspects, but healing is something that opens up your world to others'. Similarly, Margaret expressed her feeling that healing is a vocation and identity that overrides other statuses one holds: 'It's not about being a healer. You can be a secretary or a teacher or whatever but healing is a calling and it's in you, part of you. I suppose I couldn't escape it but it brings so much joy that it's OK … I don't get that joy from being an administrator'. Thus the participants reported gaining both a personal sense of importance from healing and also a positive feeling that they were contributing to others' lives, moving away from the idea that healing was something that one did to the notion that healing was a central part of what one was.

Another similarity in the women's accounts of healing was an emphasis on their own experiences of difficulty or suffering. In many ways the participants seemed to fulfil the criteria for being 'wounded healers' (Nouwen 1977): they all had some degree of poor health, from Liz who reported her health to be highly debilitating at times, to Maria who had experienced bouts of a strange muscular illness that she reported defied definition or categorisation by her GP. However, both Alex and Margaret also said they had histories of illness and/or personally difficult lives, which they accounted for as positive ways of understanding the ill health of others. For example, Alex reported: 'I saw a lot of trouble when I was young and it developed me, developed me in so many ways ... I also had domestic troubles and I was beaten quite badly ... if you take these times and use them its humbling and you understand others better when you heal'.

Within the women's narratives, being damaged by other people or experiences was reworked into experiences of growth and positive change. Healing was positively affected by personal difficulty, even ongoing personal ill health and suffering. This may be compared to some of the ethical codes of many organised CAM therapies that suggest that the therapist needs to be healthy to treat others. At the same time, the 'wounded healer' concept (seen as a positive thing for therapists to mobilise in their own lives) is found in some other therapies – especially those that are less professionally developed and which do not have well-developed ethical or professional codes of conduct (Lee-Treweek and Thomson 2005).The concept of the 'wounded healer' also echoes a common theme in anthropological studies of spirit possession and mediumship.[4]

The last point of similarity between the women that I want to draw attention to is their social positions: all four women were either lower-middle class or working class in traditional terms of occupational categorisations. They lived in Staffordshire, three in a large town and one in a village location but all in quite ordinary circumstances. As McClean (2006) has noted, there is often an association made within sociology between the middle class and New Age or folk forms of healing, the assumption being that middle class people have more time for alternative forms of healing than less wealthy individuals. However, folk knowledge of healing is often found within working-class communities and, as here, dedicated folk healers can come from working-class backgrounds and have considerable influence in sections of their communities.

Are You a Folk Healer? Descriptions and Identity

Whilst the boundaries of folk knowledge and its relationship to other forms is of interest to academics, for those who undertake healing, sometimes even the language of such discussions is foreign. A case in point was the term 'folk healing', and during the interviews I asked the participants about what the term meant to them. This term was not recognised in their self-descriptions. As Margaret commented, 'I guess it's true that I am a healer of 'folk' so I suppose I am a folk healer ... and I'm not a doctor or nurse and I wouldn't say I am a CAM healer ... Folk healer is quite a good term.' Likewise Liz commented, 'How would you describe me? Well, I just do what I do, it's natural to me now that it's more a part of me than a job or activity to do ... I wouldn't relate to the term folk healer because it's an alien idea but thinking of it I like it'. Maria, however, was less impressed,

> It doesn't sound – well, it doesn't sound very friendly. Folk healer is like folk singer, quite old fashioned and I imagine people in knitted sweaters [laughs]. But I think it's more complex than us being old fogeys who keep up old ways. I integrate new aspects as and when I find them and, I suppose, whether they complement what I do with people.

Such comments emphasise the way that the healer identity is under continual revision as well as being about 'keeping up old ways'. The interviewees preferred the singular term 'healer' as a way of describing themselves. As Alex put it: 'I think being a healer suggests you can chop and change what you do. It's not a set thing and it shouldn't be. I am always changing how I work with people and that's the interesting bit'.

From the views of the participants it could be said that the notion of the 'folk healer' is an academic construction and fairly meaningless to those it is supposed to describe. Instead, participants often chose the term healer for themselves. In this way the participants also indicated that they were healers first and foremost, not pinning themselves down to any particular mode of healing but open to using different techniques and emphasising their eclecticism. For those working in CAM, they either placed the form of healing in front (as in Reiki healer) or just used the term CAM healer.

What Do You Do to Heal People and How Do You Work?

All of the healers interviewed worked in their own homes, often in spare bedrooms, offices or converted spaces. On some occasions they all said that they worked at clients houses. Typical clients were said to be women, usually living very locally and who came for healing for a variety of long-term or chronic-health or well-being issues. Most commonly cited illnesses and symptoms were musculoskeletal pain and immobility, headaches, stress and worry or recognised mental health problems, such as depression and anxiety. The length of time spent working with a client was reported to be quite long with individual sessions lasting from an hour to an afternoon. It also seemed that the patient–healer relationship might be maintained for months or even years. Methods of healing were varied and depended on the type of healing that significant others had taught them, and their experience of, and interest in, other techniques. Margaret stated that she preferred working with energy and sometimes used stones and crystals for healing. She also believed in talking to people and helping them to harness their own power through meditation on objects of importance to them. Indeed, for all the participants pastoral care was a core component of what they felt they did for people they worked with. Maria was inspired by her mother's Italian roots and the type of folk medicine, often based on using plants, that she had taught her, but also on nutrition and food and on a variation of positive thinking. She commented:

> because of the Roman Catholic link with migrant Italians, it's not surprising that Mum did use prayer and religious practices, many of which I do not have access to as Mum died relatively young and my memory of the detail of them is quite poor. However, I am very interested in positive thinking and I use some self-hypnosis techniques which are self-taught and I can see the link with this and stuff like prayer.

Liz and Alex were perhaps the most open about the kind of modalities they deployed to help people and the process involved in this. As Liz noted:

> When someone chooses to come and see me I am very clear that I am a healer not a fixer. Orthodox medicine fixes you … healing may not do that for you and you may remain ill. But you do gain in other ways with healing like acceptance, relief from fear and recognition of being loved … I tell

> people this because I use different ways to work but they won't be fixed, the process is longer and the journey is different … My angels might work with them to deal with a problem and I might help that to happen through laying on of hands. I might also work through stones and that will often work the same way with divine intervention. I might use some muscle massage if I feel it is appropriate … I will always talk with the person and that is often the longest and most important bit.

For all of the interviewees no particular type of technique was out of bounds and they used the approach of a *bricoleur* – to use Lévi-Strauss's (1966) well-known term – in choosing what to use and when. Folk healing also provides ample opportunity for the personalising of healing techniques, the development of new ones and the modification of others. Whilst McClean (2006: 49) has also noted personalisation to be important to many CAM practitioners, one would think that for folk healers, who work completely in the private sphere as individuals and without training or any external monitoring, as having more opportunity for this type of embellishment and personalisation. But most of the techniques discussed by these women reminded me of CAM therapies, such as crystal therapy, relaxation and self-hypnosis, counselling and various energy therapies. In other words, the healers were not that different from some CAM healers in terms of what they actually did to people who chose to use them for their healing services. But the women were different in the way that they worked. For instance, they all reported that they rarely put time boundaries around what they did, so that the length of a session was dictated by the experience of healing they had with their recipient and what they perceived to be the recipient's needs. The women were also different to many CAM healers in terms of attitudes to payment and money: all of the healers reported that they asked for a 'contribution' that was decided upon by the recipient; they also noted that quite often it was not possible for the recipient to pay anything, and so they volunteered their help for free. Indeed, free treatment might continue over an extended period. This way of working is different from CAM therapists who, whilst they might have specific times when they offer 'freebies' (either as introductions to bring in new trade or through some sense of volunteering in the community), the vast majority of their work has a set fee and is undertaken to make a living.

Old Role and New Roles: Mapping Social Change through Folk Healers' Experiences

During the interviews I was concerned to find out how the healers felt their healing experiences and clientele had changed over the years as CAM had begun to professionalise. One question I asked concerned if and when they had noticed any change. All reported that they began to see changes between ten and twenty years ago, both in terms of clients and in the growing market of CAM healers:

MARIA: I began to see a lot more people advertising around [CAM practitioners] and some people who I had been working with [clients] said to me that they were trying new things. It didn't bother me to be honest at first because I do what I do and I'm not a full time person – I suppose I am an opportunist healer.

GLT: How long ago was that?

MARIA: I suppose the main change in things began in the early 1990s. All these young bucks began to get into CAM and it drew a lot of bad sorts who wanted the money but weren't bothered about the real healing part of it. You've got to remember this was just after the '80s when people got greedy and some of that greed was still about.

For Margaret, the 1990s saw the market begin to be flooded by people who she felt realised that healing was a good way to make money. Whilst she admitted CAM healers were not all bad, she did feel that the spirit of folk healing as a charitable act with poor remuneration and a community focus was somewhat lost:

> The likes of me were standing against a tide and the tide is continuing to come in ... There is something about doing for people that is lost here, everything is for a cost ... Whereas I might go to someone's house and work with them and ask for a contribution, that's thirty to forty pounds an hour to many of these CAM practitioners.

Similarly, Liz noted changes that seemed to have left her behind:

> It's hard to say when it started for sure ... I guess the mid to late 1990s was when I realised, but friends of mine started doing Reiki and other courses and not to be nasty, but they were doing it with a wish to heal but little ability and this idea came up that anyone can heal ... Anyone can do

> anything these days, give them a certificate ... You see, we don't compete, people like me, because we don't want to ... We don't do this [healing] for the same reasons [as CAM practitioners] but it's hard when you see it all changing around you.

Although such changes were noted to have started some time ago, all the healers mentioned an escalation in the number of trained healers now working in their area. As Liz notes above, in theory there is no competition between these groups because they work within their own fields of influence and with different clientele. However, as CAM therapies annex folk forms of healing and semi-professionalise them, it is unsurprising that concern was raised about the way CAM practice might be effecting folk healing.

It was interesting to note the way these women felt that the growth in CAM had affected their position or standing in their communities and society in general. 'I don't think people do look at you as having special skills necessarily now, Liz said, adding: 'A small minority will understand that you have built up knowledge over time but with the number of clowns there are going about saying, "I'm a healer" – well, it's a bit embarrassing sometimes'. Margaret agreed:

> To have the role of helping people through healing is an incredible privilege but with anyone doing it and using all kinds of therapies the balance is wrong. It's like a take away, you can have any number of types of food and types of therapy from different places, but as long as you have the piece of paper, that's OK ... Maybe some law will come in and I will be unable to do what I do now, whereas someone with the piece of paper will.

The problem of differentiating oneself from those who these women saw as inauthentic seemed to be a contemporary problem for them. Alex commented: 'How are people to know who to go to? I am lucky as people come to me through word of mouth and I like to feel that the right type of people are drawn to what I do'. Similarly, Maria noted, 'it's hard knowing how to present yourself when there is so much rubbish going on and I don't want to associate with that ... I see my healing as pure and coming from a pure heart ... I do my best for whoever comes to me and not having certificates is not important, not in my tradition it isn't'.

All the healers reported having watched CAM grow over the last decade or so and also recognised the threat this could pose to their activities, roles and status. Whilst CAM practitioners could 'evidence' their skills in a visible and contemporary fashion, these women were unable to do this. For some clients this was not a problem but for many others the kind of advice given out by groups such as the Prince of Wales Foundation for Integrated Health – that consumers should check healers' credentials and qualifications – served to indicate to potential clients that healers without these are not genuine. In other words, the contemporary patterns of professional development in CAM were felt to undermine folk healers' traditional skills and motivations for healing.

Responses to the CAM Threat: To Train or Not to Train

So far we have seen how the healers interviewed have perceived the changes in the healing marketplace around them and recognised the way that their practice is affected by the development of CAM. However, some had also begun to think about possible responses to this change and, in particular, the idea that they should train to improve their status and market position. It has to be remembered that finance is not the key issue in the work of these women, and so it is likely that they are seeking to shore up something else by training. I would argue here that they are most concerned about a loss of identity as healers. Although being genuine and authentic are key concerns for the participants, there was also a strong fear of losing their roles as healers altogether, and training would be one way of ensuring that this did not happen. Margaret, the oldest healer with the most experience, explained the dilemmas of training or not in this way:

> I am concerned about being unable to do what I love to do and what I have been born to. It's embarrassing to admit but sometimes I have looked at courses, but they are so expensive. There was one for shamanistic training on the web and based in America, but by doing that I could get insurance and cover myself ... These days you don't know if someone will complain and at present I can't get insurance ... Its worth thinking of.

Similarly, Maria had considered training:

> It's not like in my Mum's day when you could do all sorts of things ... I get less people interested now and because it's part of me [healing] it's like not

> being able to be yourself. Then again I have friends who do Reiki who are fully booked so, why not just do Reiki? A few weekends and, bingo! You are a master in no time. I spend all my life learning, watching and helping and I don't have the fancy title.

For Alex there was also an issue of pride: 'In doing a course I feel I would be moving from what I am and my heritage – and also I don't want to be seen as part of that mass of people who do a short course and heal. It doesn't work like that'.

Despite considering training, all of the healers had rejected this strategy at this point because they felt it would damage their sense of who they were, what they did, and why they did it – they saw drawbacks in the loss of their healer identity in the community. In practical terms, though, training in CAM was attractive. After training they could get insurance, they could be listed on official registers, their practice could open up to be more lucrative and they could expand the type of work they undertook. However, from their own accounts it seemed that, whilst they were resisting that way of working now, the draw of undertaking CAM training was getting stronger.

Conclusion: Interpreting the Healers' Accounts

The expansion of CAM in Britain and Ireland has massive implications for those healers who might be considered to have been 'left behind'. As Stone (2002) notes, there are over 200 CAM practitioners in the U.K., and whilst that indicates the diversity within the market there are some key shared features between many of these. Most CAMs are beginning to organise themselves and deal with issues such as regulation, setting standards in training, professional identity, ethics and values, and management of entry or the right to work within the modality. Granted, some CAMs have moved further along the road in tackling these issues than others, with the big five of osteopathy, chiropractic, medical herbalism, acupuncture and homoeopathy being the most developed in their progress and thinking. And, for some CAM groups, thinking about these issues has become so important that major splits have formed within them as they debate how to put a professional project into place. But there are indications across the board that these issues are of increasing importance. As Bowman (1999) notes, even the most esoteric CAMs are at least attempting to mimic their big five counterparts, with the idea that charismatic training should be legitimated with some combination of letters after one's name, with certificates in spiritual counselling development (and so forth) being offered, and with schools of healing springing up in New Age towns such as Totnes and Glastonbury, as well as in such seemingly less-likely spots as Luton and Falkirk. Framed by such changes, folk healing is to some extent being left as the activity of the amateur, the (very) part-timer and the individual who, for whatever reason, is unable to join a legitimate CAM. It is easy to see why the interviewees discussed here find the ever-expanding world of CAM problematic in relation to positioning themselves within the healing market.

The folk healers discussed here felt they were no longer able to exert their identities within their community as healers for all and sundry; instead, they were in the process of redefining themselves as specialist healers. Word of mouth passed on their skills and the clientele was more likely to come for special sittings. Pastoral care relationships, in which their roles were redefined as special mentoring in which healing was constituted more by relationship than by actual healing activities, seemed to be the norm. As many folk-healing activities have been 'borrowed' by CAM healing forms, folk healers have to develop their repertoire to gain market position. In particular, it seemed that pastoral care is very important to the interviewees; weakened by their inability to annex and then protect their skills, these healers were instead falling back on intense therapeutic and pastoral care relationships as the basis of what they had to offer. The empirical research showed that whilst the 'old' roles of the folk healer may be changing, the new folk healer is moving with the times to save their identity. At the same time, the interviewees appeared bitter and yearned for a reinstatement of more traditional roles, ones that they feel to be their 'natural' birthright. It seems that there is a trade-off between traditional authenticity and what needs to be done to ensure the continuance of folk community healing.

However, the interviewees demonstrate that they are able to fight back and resist notions that they are losing out to the processes of social change that are happening around healing in the U.K. By mobilising ideas about authenticity and biography, they can make claims to their clientele and communities about having legitimacy as healers. It is also the case that their kinds of claims are likely to be appealing to particular types of clients. Whilst many people using forms of healing outside orthodox or conventional arenas will be influenced by evidence that a practitioner has been trained in some professional capacity, there are likely to be others who find practitioners who work outside these boundaries more appealing. Given also that we know that initial referral mainly comes from word of mouth recommendation by kin and friends, or (in some cases) curiosity (Lee-Treweek 2002), folk healers may still have some special 'pulling power' when it comes to gaining clients. Folk healers are also, if one can believe their own accounts, deeply embedded in the communities around them (see Chapter 3, this volume). Indeed, they are so embedded that finding them to interview is very difficult (see also Chapter 4, this volume): they do not advertise in conventional CAM environments and they do not necessarily use CAM settings – like mind, body and spirit festivals and fairs – for self promotion. Again, it is word of mouth that is the best mechanism for revealing their presence because their work is undertaken alone and they work as individuals.

The accounts of the interviewees were highly critical of other people working within CAM, particularly with regard to their motives and natural abilities. The participants used a range of ways to demonstrate the inappropriateness of some individuals working within CAM, including critiquing systems of payment, and there are a number of ways this can be interpreted. On the one hand, it is easy to see these healers' criticisms about payment for healing and the flooding of the market with CAM practitioners as a disgruntled response to their loss of a market niche. However, it is does not seem to me a convincing argument that these concerns are about financial loss as these healers do not operate within the same system of payment for healing as most CAM practitioners; instead, they present themselves as community workers, addressing needs deep in the heart of their locales. Whilst this account is compelling I cannot help but consider the idea, from the empirical evidence, that the women interviewed might be getting more from their position as healers than their recipients. They reported working in jobs they found relatively dull in comparison to their healing activities, whereas healing brought them into contact with a range of different people who they worked with for fairly lengthy periods of time. Healing therefore provided another outlet for identity and also a chance to be important to other people.

The issue of healing and identity is crucially important to the participants, particularly the notion that current circumstances represent a threat to their identity. Here we have four women who maintain that they have been healers from birth, or at least from early on in their lives, and it would be very difficult for someone in that position to accept training. In a sense, the healers' identities and narratives have been bound up with the idea that they are born to do this work and that it is birth, not training, that gives them a unique healing ability. To backtrack from this position into accepting training takes a complete reframing of what their lives have been about: their biographies; their relationships to other healers in their families; their relationships with people they provide healing services to; and their sense of motivation to heal. Even their critiques of other healers fall apart if they themselves join the mass of CAM practitioners and take up the ways of working expected within a particular CAM modality. In other words, such a leap of identity is not easily made. Their resistance to CAM healing, and with it their narratives of authenticity and their promotion of their 'real healing' over other forms, also creates a sense of being special and being someone who is valued within the sectors of the community that they work with. Psychologically, the interviewees were in a precarious position in which they had much to lose if they withdrew from their roles as folk healers.

It is pertinent to ask what will happen to this type of healer in the future. What is clear is that, for now, these women will remain community-based untrained healers. However, one wonders about their ability to pass on their skills to others in their families. For some of the interviewees there are no younger people to influence towards folk healing, and for others one has to wonder what value their children will place on folk healing within a climate where qualification and training is the premier route to legitimacy in healing. At the same time, some of the healers themselves seemed reluctantly drawn to CAM training, and whilst they were negative about the idea, it was clear they had spent considerable time thinking through the issues. Lay healing in the domestic home will always exist; however, whether folk healers as a community resource will continue to exist remains to be seen.

Notes

1. Source: Professor Kim Burton, osteopath (personal communication, July 2000).
2. See Chapter 10 (this volume) for a discussion of the legal status of folk and CAM healers.
3. The participants have been given pseudonyms and identifying details have been altered to protect their anonymity.
4. See also Chapter 7 (this volume) on crystal and spiritual healers.

References

Bakx, K. 1991. 'The "Eclipse" of Folk Medicine in Western Society', *Sociology of Health And Illness* 13: 20–38.

Bowman, M. 1999. 'Healing in the Spiritual Marketplace', *Social Compass* 46(2): 181–89.

Cant, S. and U. Sharma. 1998. 'Reflexivity, Ethnography and the Professions (Complementary Medicine): Watching You Watching Me Watching You (And Writing About Both Of Us)', *Sociological Review* 46(2): 244–63.

Chamberlain, M. 1981. *Old Wives Tales*. London: Virago.

Helman, C. 2006. *Suburban Shaman: Tales From Medicine's Frontline*. London: Hammersmith Press.

Lee-Treweek, G. 2002. 'Trust In Complementary and Alternative Medicine: The Case of Cranial Osteopathy', *Sociological Review* 50(1): 31–49.

Lee-Treweek, G. and H. Thomson. 2005. 'Accora the Healer: Deception and Fraudulent Identity in Healing', in G. Lee-Treweek, T. Heller, S. Spurr, H. Macqueen and J. Katz (eds), *Perspectives On Complementary And Alternative Medicine: A Reader*. London: Routledge.

Lévi-Strauss, C. 1966. *The Savage Mind*. London: Weidenfeld And Nicholson.

McClean, S. 2006. *An Ethnography Of Crystal And Spiritual Healers In Northern England: Marginal Medicine And Mainstream Concerns*. New York: Edwin Mellen Press.

May, W.F. 1997. 'Money and the Medical Profession', *Kennedy Institute Of Ethics Journal* 7(1): 1–13.

Nicholls, P. 1988. *Homeopathy And The Medical Profession*. London: Croom Helm.

Nouwen, H. 1977. *The Wounded Healer*. New York: Doubleday.
Saks, M. 1996. 'From Quackery to Complementary Medicine: The Shifting Boundaries between Orthodox and Unorthodox Medical Knowledge', in S. Cant and U. Sharma (eds), *Complementary And Alternative Medicines: Knowledge In Practice*. London: Free Association Books.
______. 2004. 'Political and Historical Perspectives', in T. Heller, G. Lee-Treweek, J. Katz, J. Stone and S. Spurr (eds), *Perspectives On Complementary And Alternative Medicine*. London: Routledge.
Stone, J. 2002. *An Ethical Framework For Complementary And Alternative Therapists*. London: Routledge.
Twigg, J. 2000. *Bathing, The Body And Community Care*. London: Routledge.
______. 2003. 'The Body and Bathing: Help with Personal Care at Home', in C.A. Faircloth (ed.) *Ageing Bodies: Images and Everyday Experiences*. Walnut Creek, CA: Altamira Press.
Wing, D.M. 1998. 'A Comparison of Traditional Folk Healing Concepts with Contemporary Healing Concepts', *Journal of Community Health Nursing* 15(3): 143–54.

Chapter 10

Beyond Legislation: Why Chicken Soup and Regulation Don't Mix

Julie Stone

Introduction

Folk healing in Britain has, with the exception of herbal medicine, been largely excluded from the realm of state regulation.[1] This chapter will explore why this has been the case and the ongoing feasibility of this situation, at a time when healthcare regulation purports to have moved away from professional self-interest towards a framework based predominantly on patient safety. Current developments include a major overhaul of the regulation of conventional healthcare practitioners,[2] and a significant professionalisation within complementary and alternative medicine (CAM), including funding from the U.K. government to help develop improved systems of CAM voluntary self-regulation.[3]

Having considered the debates surrounding classification and nomenclature, arguments for and against more formal regulation of folk medicine will be reviewed by comparing and contrasting folk medicine first with CAM (given apparent similarities and overlap between the two phenomena), and then with conventional medicine, to the extent that healers, like conventional practitioners, claim that they are able to provide relief from sickness and disease.

Two polarised positions will be considered: pro-regulation and anti-regulation. The principal pro-regulation argument is based on the assertion that any person holding themselves out as a healer should be regulated on the basis of public protection, albeit that the scientific efficacy and effectiveness of folk healing cannot be conventionally assessed. Failure to regulate, it is argued, exposes users of folk medicine to an unacceptable level of risk of harm from potentially unskilled and unsafe practitioners. A secondary argument is that the unregulated and unaffiliated status of folk healers also sits uncomfortably alongside the increasing regulation and professionalisation of CAM. The anti-regulation arguments are more diverse but turn, largely, on the non-professionalised status of many folk healers, which makes it hard, if not impossible, to set and maintain consistent standards; they also rest on the nature of the therapies being offered, which, by virtue of sitting outside a biomedical framework, are not subject to 'scientific' validation and, arguably, may not be amenable to regulation. This chapter will evaluate arguments for and against each of these positions. Whilst concluding that folk healing sits uneasily with formal regulation, it will, nonetheless, recommend licensing folk healers as a model of regulation which could enhance public safety without fettering the rights of individuals to practise and seek therapies of their choosing.

Statutory Regulation and its Public Protection Rationale

Doctors, nurses and other conventional healthcare practitioners are regulated by statute. Various, high profile scandals have prompted a radical overhaul of the regulation of health professions. Proposals for reform have attempted to counter criticisms that regulation has been overly dominated by professional self-interest, at the expense of public protection and stakeholder involvement (Walshe and Benson 2005). A long-awaited White Paper on the regulation of health professionals sets out the principles which underpin statutory regulation, stressing the public interest rationale:

> [T]here are a number of key principles that should underpin statutory professional regulation.
>
> First, its overriding interest should be the safety and quality of the care that patients receive from health professionals.
>
> Second, professional regulation needs to sustain the confidence of both the public and the professions through demonstrable impartiality.

Regulators need to be independent of government, the professionals themselves, employers, educators and all the other interest groups involved in healthcare.

Third, professional regulation should be as much about sustaining, improving and assuring the professional standards of the overwhelming majority of health professionals as it is about identifying and addressing poor practice or bad behaviour.

Fourth, professional regulation should not create unnecessary burdens, but be proportionate to the risk it addresses and the benefit it brings.

Finally, we need a system that ensures the strength and integrity of health professionals within the United Kingdom, but is sufficiently flexible to work effectively for the different health needs and healthcare approaches within and without the NHS in England, Scotland, Wales and Northern Ireland and to adapt to future changes' (DoH 2007: 8).

The Current Regulatory Status of CAM and Folk Healing

Compared to the intensive regulation of conventional healthcare practitioners, many CAM practitioners and most folk healers operate outside formal systems of regulation. Whilst all CAM practitioners and folk healers are subject to common law – meaning that they can, theoretically, be sued for assault, negligence, or breach of contract (if they offer their services on a contractual basis) – as well as being subject to criminal laws as ordinary citizens, their ability to set up in practice as healers requires no licence or formal qualifications, and they are free to offer healing services without even rudimentary checks as to their background, character or competence.

This does not mean that folk healers are entirely free from regulation. Formal regulation is but one mechanism for regulating behaviour, albeit one which is highly valorised in Ireland and the U.K.'s biomedically orientated healthcare system. All healers self-regulate to the extent that they moderate their own conduct and practice in accordance with societal norms and expectations. Hopefully, folk healers are motivated by their client's interests, and practise within the limits of their competence and with healing intent. Indeed, within traditional healing cultures, the lengthy process of apprenticeship required before healers are allowed to practise autonomously includes substantial training on the ethical dimensions of practice, albeit outside the strictures of a formalised, and externally accredited, curriculum.

Therapists and healers who charge money for their services are, additionally, subject to market forces, to the extent that if they fail to provide what is perceived to be an adequate service, or if they make claims which exceed their capabilities, then their reputation will be lost and their client base (depending on the available competition) is likely to dry up.[4] Folk healers may, additionally, lose the confidence of their community if their healing ministrations repeatedly fail, and face being ostracised if they behave unethically or inappropriately.

Voluntary versus Statutory Regulation

The regulatory context of CAM in the U.K. is, for the main part, one of voluntary self-regulation. Systems of voluntary self-regulation range from loose affiliations of individuals to highly formalised systems of registration and fitness to practise. The main differences between a voluntary and statutory system are as follows:

> Ideally, an effective voluntary self-regulating scheme will share many of the features of professionally-led statutory regulation, namely: a single register of practitioners per profession; externally accredited education and training; codes of ethics; and FTP processes/complaints mechanisms. The key difference in terms of public protection is that a voluntary system lacks statutory protection of title. What this means is that people who are not on a register may nonetheless practise a regulated therapy or use a particular title without that constituting a criminal offence.... Professionally led statutory regulation creates a protected title, and in a few cases, protected functions, which are limited to professionals on a statutory register. (Stone 2005a: 18)

Whereas CAM was highly fragmented in the past, many CAM therapies are now moving towards professionalisation, coming together under single registers per profession, standardising their training and qualification requirements, and adopting formal complaints processes.

Osteopathy and chiropractic are, somewhat anomalously, statutorily regulated in the UK.[5] The awarding of statutory status to these two professions – widely perceived by the public, if not by the professions themselves, to be part of CAM – created a climate of expectation amongst other professionally well-organised CAM therapies that statutory regulation would be forthcoming to other

CAM disciplines in due course (Stone 2005b). This expectation was based, in part, on a view of regulation as predominantly being a mechanism to provide status and ensure occupational advantage through a system of professional closure. Indeed, the original legislation governing osteopathy and chiropractic explicitly gave their respective regulatory body a role in promoting the profession, a role which is now recognised to sit uncomfortably with the overarching duty of a modern healthcare regulatory body to protect the public.[6]

It would, however, be specious to pretend that statutory regulation does not raise the profile of an occupational group, which is presumably why some CAM therapies still hope to pursue statutory, rather than voluntary, regulation. The description of regulation as a mechanism for enhancing a profession's reputation is evident in a consultation on federal regulation which, having discussed the patient safety rationale for regulation, goes on to state:

> The fundamental reason for regulation is the safeguarding of the public, but there are other benefits to individual practitioners and the profession as a whole. The status of practitioners is enhanced as a result of improved standards across the profession. Reputation is protected from the work of bogus practitioners who would be prevented from registering with a regulatory body. Practitioners are able to demonstrate that they are working to agreed codes for the profession as a whole, which can act as a protection against allegations. They can also demonstrate to statutory and private health providers that they are meeting the requirements of the regulatory body. (Jack 2006)

The document continues by citing social historian, Walter Wardwell:

> In addition to the concern for the public's welfare and for the guild-type benefits which all professions seek for their members, a new profession primarily wants official recognition legitimising its work. This not only helps attract clients but it confers legal standing on the profession with all the rights and privileges pertaining thereto. (ibid.)

The status and privilege arguments raised were no doubt intended to win over practitioners who continued to be wary of regulation. The language sits uncomfortably, however, with current regulatory rhetoric, which stresses professional responsibilities over professional privilege, in an attempt to provide public reassurance that healthcare regulation does not involve cosy clubs of practitioners protecting their own. In any event, the pursuit by CAM of enhanced 'status' via statutory regulation has been singularly unsuccessful. The current Labour government has promoted 'light touch regulation', attempting to reduce the overall regulatory burden wherever possible.[7] It has sought to achieve this by cutting 'red tape' and reducing administrative and inspection burdens, putting in place systems of regulation which are 'risk-based' and commensurate to the activity in question.[8] In this political climate, the government has viewed the regulation of small therapies on a therapy-by-therapy basis as antithetical, promoting the merger of regulated healthcare professions under federal, or umbrella, bodies.[9]

Largely in reliance of an influential House of Lords Select Committee report (House of Lords 2000), the current government has accepted the view that voluntary self-regulation provides sufficient safeguards for patients accessing the majority of CAM therapies. To this end, it has supported moves towards voluntary self-regulation in the CAM sector, limiting statutory regulation at the current time to acupuncture and herbal medicine (adding traditional Chinese medicine – TCM – as a third and distinct entity, in seeming contradiction of the House of Lord's recommendations, which had placed TCM in a category of long-established therapies which could not be explained within biomedical paradigms and did not, in the Select Committee's view, require statutory regulation).

To date, regulation of folk medicine has been singularly absent from wider debates regarding regulation of CAM in the U.K. Indeed, when the House of Lords' Select Committee considered complementary and alternative therapies, many of the healing traditions being considered within this volume – such as crystal therapy (see Chapter 6), as well as dowsing, radionics, iridology, and kinesiology – fell within a category (3b) seen as 'lacking any credible evidence base' and 'indifferent to the scientific principles of conventional medicine' (House of Lords Summary of Recommendations). These therapies were distinguished from other long-established and traditional systems of healthcare, such as Ayurvedic medicine and TCM (category 3a). Whereas these longer established therapies were granted a degree of respect and credibility, therapies in the 3b category were all but dismissed out of hand:

> Some CAM therapies, and especially those in the Group 3a, have very specific philosophies that have evolved over centuries of use. Often these

> have developed into views about how the body functions and how disease is caused. Sometimes these are linked to the dominant religious philosophies of their country of origin. Examples include Ayurvedic medicine, and Traditional Chinese medicine. However, there is no established evidence base supporting these. The lack of an evidence base is even more evident in the case of those therapies we classify in Group 3b, and these must be subject to rigorous appraisal. Many conventional medical scientists, while accepting the validity of accumulative empirical observation, believe that those therapeutic disciplines that are based principally on abstract philosophy and not on scientific reasoning and experiment have little place in medicine. (ibid.)

The House of Lords perpetuated two challengeable concepts. The first was that regulation of health professions was a privilege to be 'earned' by 'respectable' CAM therapies, and the second was that integration 'into' conventional medicine required an established evidence base, a position which has hampered attempts to commission CAM services within the NHS and which ignores the value placed by patients on therapies such as healing and homeopathy where these have been provided on the NHS. Nonetheless, this Report probably accounts for why folk medicine has sat, and continues to sit, outside formal regulatory structures.

The House of Lords's arguments are sharply at odds with contemporary rhetoric, which sees the regulation of professionals as being a mechanism to protect patients through the setting and maintenance of high, professional standards. Whereas regulation of CAM therapies in the past might have required endorsement by the medical establishment, such 'approval' should no longer be seen as dictating whether CAM, or indeed folk healing, ought to be regulated on the basis of public protection. Arguably, the House of Lords's three-fold grouping now looks decidedly dated. Indeed, public protection, it will be argued, is more of a concern in precisely those therapies which lack professional organisation, and where individuals are more or less free to practise without any external constraint.

Whilst folk healers may be highly visible in their communities, they are largely overlooked in strategic debates around professionalisation, standards-setting and education. This may be because healers in Britain tend to work as individuals and not as part of a collective or wider occupational group. Folk healers may individually reject the role of 'health professional' and/or belong to organisations whose practitioners collectively eschew formal regulation, which they believe would compromise their holistic style of practice. The standardisation and consistency which professionalisation presupposes may sit ill with the charismatic and individualistic nature of some healers, and some healing traditions.

The position of folk healing in Britain and Ireland is somewhat different to the view of traditional healing held by the World Health Organisation (WHO). The WHO defines traditional medicine (TM) in the following terms: 'Traditional medicine is the sum total of the knowledge, skills, and practices based on the theories, beliefs, and experiences indigenous to different cultures, whether explicable or not, used in the maintenance of health as well as in the prevention, diagnosis, improvement or treatment of physical and mental illness' (WHO 2000: 1).

The WHO notes that countries in Africa, Asia and Latin America use TM to help meet some of their primary healthcare needs. In Africa, up to 80 per cent of the population uses TM for primary healthcare. The WHO view traditional healing as falling very much within a potential regulatory remit (WHO 2002). This is perhaps not surprising, given that in many parts of the world, traditional or folk healing constitutes a significant part of overall healthcare delivery,[10] unlike folk healing in Ireland and the U.K., where the biomedical model of health predominates and folk healing operates very much at the margins. In such countries, adaptations of TM and folk healing are termed 'complementary' or 'alternative' (see Chapter 8, this volume).

Nomenclature and Definitions

In other chapters in this volume, various definitions of folk healing have been advanced (see Chapter 1 and Chapter 8). One way of defining folk traditions would be by means of exclusion; namely, to define folk healing as encompassing the broad range of native and indigenous healing practices which are practised outside formal healthcare systems, and are not seen as being part of CAM. Such a definition would certainly be in keeping with definitions of CAM, which have in the past defined CAM as that which is excluded from conventional or orthodox medicine.

Perhaps a more defining feature of folk healing, however, is the extent to which it has remained outside economically defined and commercially orientated healthcare systems, and has, to date, significantly resisted commoditisation. For these reasons, Eskinazi's definition might be more apposite:

> alternative medicine [may] be defined as a broad set of health care practices (i.e. already available to the public) that are not readily integrated into the dominant health care model, because they pose challenges to diverse societal beliefs and practices (cultural, economic, scientific, medical, and educational). This definition brings into focus factors that may play a major role in the a priori acceptance or rejection of various alternative health care practices by any society. Unlike criteria of current definitions, those of the proposed definition would not be expected to change significantly without significant societal changes. (Eskinazi 1998: 1622)

Such a definition certainly seems to capture the 'otherness' of folk healing, a set of practices which somewhat stubbornly, and quite possibly deliberately, elude formal processes of professionalisation and regulation.

Nomenclature within CAM has clearly been a highly contested issue. The transition from 'fringe', 'unconventional', 'alternative', 'complementary and alternative', to 'integrated medicine' – the newest term – says much about CAM's relative fortunes compared to hegemonic orthodox medicine, and little about the substance of the modalities in question. Ironically, the use of the term 'traditional medicine', now firmly associated with native, indigenous healing rather than biomedical scientific practice, could be seen as squaring the circle, acknowledging the plurality of healing methods that co-exist in today's global and globalised healing environment. Bound up within categorisations and groupings are complex debates about legitimacy, authenticity and, ultimately, power – in this context, the power for healers to call themselves what they like, to practise such healing techniques as they see fit, and to do so free from external constraint beyond community and client-based approval or censure.

Paradoxically, therapies which could be described as folk or traditional healing in their place of origin, and which have been imported into the U.K. (and professionalised and commoditised), such as traditional Chinese herbal medicine (TCHM), are very much seen as part of CAM. Indeed, TCHM in particular occupies a visible place on the high street and is moving towards formal statutory regulation, along with acupuncture and herbal medicine. Although both British folk healing practices and TCHM may, intrinsically, approach healing in similar ways, the difference in their status is marked.

In order to examine this apparent dichotomy, Figure 10.1 looks at some of the features which folk medicine and CAM have in common, and some of the features which distinguish them. These also need to be contrasted with conventional medicine.

Professionalism, Knowledge and Legitimacy

In earlier chapters, a number of key questions have been discussed. Who is a folk healer? What claims to expertise are required to adopt the title 'healer'? Are the skills of healers learned through a process of apprenticeship or are they bestowed as a birthright? How do healers heal, and using what 'tools'? Can healing phenomena be understood within conventional scientific frameworks? If not, what belief systems underpin the basis for effectiveness of such healing systems, for both the healer and the healed? The responses to these questions yield a wide array of beliefs, customs and practices, some of which can be accommodated within a biomedical understanding of health and disease, some of which cannot.

Much of the regulation debate turns on whether the knowledge that folk healers have can properly be described as 'expert' as distinct from lay. This is because healthcare regulation has, historically, ring-fenced and delineated the activities of 'professionals' and provided occupational advantage to those who possess expert knowledge, prohibiting others, in the case of statutory regulation, from working as, or otherwise holding themselves out as, practitioners who possess such skills. Part of the difficulty in deciding where, if anywhere, folk healing should sit on a regulatory spectrum is that folk healers do not necessarily make claims of exclusivity, nor do they necessarily define themselves, or wish to be sought by others, as professionals with expert, specialised knowledge.

Table 10.1: Comparisons of Folk Healing, CAM and Conventional Healthcare in the U.K.

Folk Healing	**CAM**	**Conventional Healthcare**
Unregulated	Partially regulated	Intensely regulated
Unlicensed practitioners and products, including common foodstuffs	Voluntarily licensed practitioners, statutory licensed products (aromatherapy oils, herbal medicine products and nutritional supplements)	Statutorily regulated professionals. Statutorily regulated products (including prescription only medications)
Individually determined standards	Nationally determined standards (increasingly)	EU and internationally determined standards
No state provision	Minimal state provision via National Health Service (although growing interface via practice-based commissioning)	State provision, free at the point of delivery under auspices of National Health Services
Predominantly sole practitioners working outside formalised health systems	Sole practitioners, but increasing interface with doctors and other conventional practitioners	Part of multi-disciplinary teams of professionals trained within a formalised healthcare setting
Practitioners may or may not charge for services, or may accept payment in kind	Practitioners mostly charge for payments on a fee-paying basis (may operate sliding scale)	NHS terms and conditions nationally set. May, in addition, operate private practice at market rates.
Therapeutic practices largely irreconcilable with biomedical model	Some 'complementary' practices seen as understandable within biomedical framework, other 'alternative' practices less so, but subject, increasingly, of research (including within biomedical sector) to determine efficacy	Therapeutic practices dominated by biomedical model, with significant emphasis on evidence-based practice
Weak scientific evidence base	Emerging evidence base for some, but by no means all therapies	Strong commitment towards evidence-based practice

Chicken Soup: An Analogy

To help illustrate some of these points, let us look at chicken soup a culturally specific healing intervention used in Jewish communities within Ireland and the U.K.

It is widely accepted within Ashkenazi Jewish communities that chicken soup, sometimes referred to as 'kosher penicillin', has significant healing properties. This clear broth – made from the bones of a chicken, boiled on a stove top with onions, carrots, celery, *kneidlach* (dumplings) and other (secret) ingredients – is believed to have a beneficial effect on respiratory diseases, nervous conditions and most diseases of childhood.

Chicken soup tends to be made and dispensed by the matriarch of a household following a recipe passed down to her by her mother, and by her mother before her. Mothers traditionally initiate their daughters into the ways of chicken soup before they marry so that they can make their own chicken soup and, in time, pass the recipe on to their own daughters. By the time girls have a 'formal' chicken soup lesson, they are likely to have watched the pre-Sabbath cooking of chicken soup for many years and may even have had a subordinate role in its preparation, such as chopping the vegetables.

Over the years, chicken soup has acquired a nigh-on mythical status within the Ashkenazi Jewish diaspora and beyond. Notably, both makers and recipients believe absolutely in the healing powers of chicken soup. Chicken soup made by one's mother or grandmother is especially potent and a key 'ingredient' is the loving intent with which chicken soup is made. Whilst chicken soup can be bought in packet form ('over the counter'), this is widely felt to be a pale imitation of 'real' chicken soup, lacking the therapeutic powers of home made chicken soup.

Several points can usefully be made at this juncture. Chicken soup has not been the subject of formal 'medical' research, so is chicken soup a medicine, and are makers of chicken soup 'healers'? Certainly, lack of proof has in no sense diminished adherents' belief in its healing properties. Unlike pharmaceutical medicines, there is no standardised recipe for chicken soup. No recipe could capture the nuanced seasoning which each chicken soup-maker will assess to be 'just right'. The skills of chicken soup making are acquired over many years, one might say through a process of apprenticeship. Are chicken soup makers born into this role? Certainly, a significant proportion of Ashkenazi women will continue the tradition, although this is not to say others cannot learn how to make 'authentic' chicken soup. The making of chicken soup is not a regulated activity: making it for one's family or members of one's community requires no formal licence (unless sold commercially), and claims for its efficacy are internalised within a specific community.

The research issue has interesting ramifications for folk healing more widely. A clinical trial could be designed, for the sake of argument, to compare Mrs Cohen's chicken soup with Mrs Levy's, but questions of comparative efficacy may be of little value to the community in question. External ratings or approval will be of little interest, given that the recipients of each woman's soup will be enculturated to prefer the taste of, and derive maximum benefit from, the soup they are most familiar with. Another potential research trial might compare the relative efficacy of chicken soup against (non-kosher) beef tea, a meat-based beverage given to invalids in similar circumstances. But again, the culturally specific demand for one healing potion over another means that the results of such a trial would be of limited value. A final question at this point is whether doctors and the wider health community should be exploring whether chicken soup does, indeed, have properties so special as to merit knowledge and dissemination into the wider community. This also raises a germane question: Were chicken soup to be discovered to be the great panacea many believe it to be, who would patent it? Who would commercially manufacture it? Would its essence be lost in the process of commoditisation? These are important considerations for healing traditions considering entering the healthcare marketplace.

This example has focused on a healing remedy, rather than the healer themselves. It is also important to think about folk healers and their values and aspirations, as the question of regulation may have more to do with the status of the healer, and the relationship they have with the person seeking a cure, than the techniques they employ. Specifically, the notion of folk healers as lay people, trained and embedded within specific cultures, and committed to empowering and improving the health of the community they serve, may provide more of a clue as to why folk healing remains an unregulated phenomenon. Vickers and Heller describe folk medicine as 'health advice dispensed by a person's friends and family who do not practise a recognised health profession' (Vickers and Heller 2005: 297). They note that the way in which folk medicine is used usually has a strong relationship to a person's beliefs and accounts of health.

The key distinction as to why CAM is increasingly subject to regulation and folk medicine is not turns, principally, on the question of professionalisation. Professionalisation relates both to the person offering services and the nature of services being offered. In terms of who is offering services, Vickers and Heller describe the differences between CAM and folk medicine in the following terms:

> CAM is generally associated with defined groups of health practitioners: individuals who identify themselves as herbalists, chiropractors, Alexander teachers, and so on. Currently, folk medicine in developed western societies is generally not associated with health professionals.... In some cases, certain individuals do practise a form of folk medicine as a professional, but they are not organised into recognised professional bodies. (ibid.: 298).

In terms of the nature of the services being offered, Vickers and Heller argue that CAM comprises 'codified and recognised bodies of knowledge and expertise' (ibid.: 298). This knowledge is documented in texts that seek to guide practice. In contrast, they state: 'Folk medicine beliefs exist in vernacular (usually oral) culture, do not have established core principles, and are neither systematically interrelated nor codified' (ibid.: 298).

As previously intimated, the boundaries between conventional medicine, CAM and folk medicine are in constant flux. A number of the folk practices described in this book are currently in the process of professionalisation and at some future point are likely to be described as CAM rather than folk medicine.

Pro-Regulation Arguments

This section will explore some of the arguments in favour of more formalised regulation for folk healers. The dominant view of regulation, as stated, is patient and public protection. Regulation, it is argued, enables patients to make informed choices as to who is a respectable practitioner and who is not, which is empowering.

Safety and Quality Assurance of Folk Remedies

Some, but not all, folk healers rely on herbs and potions to induce a cure. In the U.K. and elsewhere, medicinal products are subject to strict regimes of control and licensing. Traditional and herbal remedies are regulated by statute.[11] These are in place to ensure safety, consistency and quality, notwithstanding doubts within the scientific community as to their efficacy and effectiveness. Concerns have been expressed that formulations used in traditional medicine, particularly imported traditional herbal medicines, may be unsafe because they are of dubious quality or because their consistency cannot be guaranteed, or because of mislabelling. The WHO has highlighted some of these concerns:

> Unregulated or inappropriate use of traditional medicines and practices can have negative or dangerous effects. For instance, the herb "Ma Huang" (Ephedra) is traditionally used in China to treat respiratory congestion. In the United States, the herb was marketed as a dietary aid, whose over dosage led to at least a dozen deaths, heart attacks and strokes. In Belgium, at least 70 people required renal transplant or dialysis for interstitial fibrosis of the kidney after taking a herbal preparation made from the wrong species of plant as slimming treatment. (WHO 2003)

Whereas it may be possible to regulate medicinal herbal products used by folk healers, the regulation of ordinary foodstuffs, such as garlic, or combinations of food stuffs (such as advocating spicy foods to keep colds at bay) may be harder to accommodate.[12] Food law in the U.K. includes a prohibition on claims to treat, prevent or cure disease, although it is highly likely that some healers do recommend patients eat or refrain from eating certain foods.

Safety and Quality Assurance of Folk Healers

Modern healthcare regulation is primarily concerned with public protection and public reassurance. To the extent that folk healers are making claims about their ability to cure or heal people of their ailments, they create a level of expectation in those to whom they offer services: expectations that they know what they are doing, and have reason to believe in the efficacy of what they offer. Critically, the argument in favour of more formal regulation of any practitioner who offers healing services does not depend on external proof of evidence or efficacy. Rather, the argument rests on the fact that the person is holding themselves out as a healer. In so doing, that person is creating both ethical expectations on the part of a prospective patient (that the person has skills, and will deploy them in the patient's best interests), and also, potentially, legal expectations (with or without the existence of a formal contract) that the person offering treatment owes the patient a duty of care, and may be found to be in breach of that duty should their actions fall short of an acceptable standard and cause a patient harm.[13]

Arguably, there is a much greater need to ensure the quality, safety and good faith of practitioners who work in unregulated environments, often out of their own homes, in sole, private practice, and without the supervision of colleagues or mentors found in state-provided healthcare systems. A potential safeguard, it could be argued, is that a certain level of scrutiny of healers is provided by the community itself. The extent to which this contention is viable or verifiable is questionable. In Britain and Ireland, this position may have pertained historically, when, for example, a village may have had only one expert, perhaps a 'wise woman' or 'cunning man', who had use of traditional herbs and remedies. It may still be a position which pertains within certain ethnic groups within Britain and Ireland, including immigrant populations who may continue to rely on culturally familiar remedies (see Chapter 8, this volume). But to the extent that the majority of folk healers now offer services in a crowded, pluralistic health marketplace, it may be harder for the community in which they are based to reassure or be reassured about an individual's skills, authenticity or safety.

Similarities Between Folk Healers and CAM Practitioners Requires Folk Healers to be Formally Regulated

As has been seen from the earlier discussion on nomenclature, whether a folk healer calls themselves a folk healer, a spiritual healer, a holistic therapist, or a CAM practitioner may be somewhat arbitrary. It would seem anomalous if, for the sake of argument, a kinesiologist or iridologist, given that professional bodies for these therapies exist, is regarded in a different regulatory position by dint of holding themselves out as a folk healer, rather than a CAM practitioner.

Such is the nature of voluntary self-regulation, however, that even where professional associations and registers do exist (and notably, in less professionalised therapies, a multitude of professional organisations tend to co-exist) a practitioner cannot be forced to affiliate themselves with that body, or be bound by its rules and codes of conduct. Voluntary systems vary from loose affiliations of practitioners coming together in an interest group, to highly formalised systems of regulation, including quasi-judicial disciplinary systems. But all voluntary systems rely heavily on the principle of caveat emptor ('let the buyer beware'), placing responsibility on the patient to ensure that the person they consult has appropriate skills, registration and indemnity insurance in place in case something goes wrong.

Anti-Regulation Arguments

This section will explore some of the arguments against more formalised regulation for folk healers, or against forms of regulation which replicate those designed with biomedical professions in mind.

Consumer Choice Arguments

A significant argument against formal regulation concentrates less on folk healers and the services they offer, and more on the right of consumers to opt for therapies of their own choosing from competing healthcare providers.[14] Patients, it has been argued, should be able to choose whatever form of healing they wish. This argument is made persuasively in a landmark Irish report on regulation, which notes: 'It is for the consumer to make the choice of which therapy they intend to use. Whether they wish to consult a qualified therapist such as a homeopath or an acupuncturist, a healer, the seventh son of a seventh son, a person reputed to have a cure for a particular ailment or a person with a special skill with bones; the choice is theirs' (National Working Group 2005: 7).

Critics of consumer choice point out that sick people are not in the position of ordinary consumers. The fact that patients are sick makes them vulnerable and open to exploitation, and this, it is said, requires external intervention to ensure that healers who offer treatment have appropriate skills and can be held to account if they act inappropriately, or cause a patient harm. The weakness of the free market argument is that even its most ardent advocates might accept the need for minimalist intervention to ensure that known fraudsters, convicted sex offenders and murderers are prohibited from setting themselves up as practitioners. This may militate in favour of a light-touch form of regulation, involving, for example, licensing practitioners and premises, which we will consider in the concluding section.

The consumer choice argument, in turn, has been criticised for infantilising all sick people as vulnerable, and denying them the opportunity to exercise their autonomy, including making potentially bad or ill-advised choices and wasting their money. Ironically, this potentially paternalistic argument usually comes from doctors on the basis that if patients had been better advised they would have made a wise choice to see a medically qualified practitioner who might have been able to treat them more successfully.

Inappropriateness for Folk Healing of Formal, Professionally Led Regulation

Arguably, folk healing is not amenable to formal regulation of the kind which currently regulates conventional health practitioners and is increasingly used as a model upon which to base the voluntary self-regulation of CAM therapies. This is not to say that folk healers should be entirely unregulated, but it is an argument against the dominant model of professionally led regulation in Ireland and the U.K. This form of regulation gives a profession a significant say in determining its entry standards and educational requirements, its scopes of practice, its standards of conduct, and its power to make decisions about who is and is not fit to practise.[15]

Central to the notion of professionally led regulation is the existence of a profession. Professional regulation requires there to be a body of practitioners being regulated, who share a coherent body of knowledge, ascribe to broadly similar norms of conduct and practice and whose knowledge systems are codified, transmissible, and reproducible (albeit in a state of constant development).

The obvious question is whether folk healers are professionals and whether their techniques constitute a profession. It is not possible to give a fixed answer to these questions. Relevant factors include whether the characteristics of an individual or a group of individuals bear sufficient similarity to other occupational groups treated as professionals. It is not just about how practitioners see themselves, but it is also to do with how healers are perceived by others. As certain traditions become more formalised and professionalised, they will inevitably become subject to a more intense regulatory gaze.

The Ontario Model: An Alternative Statutory Approach

An alternative to the British model of professional regulation is that adopted in Ontario, Canada, where specific healing acts are regulated in addition to professional titles.[16] An explicit scope of practice is defined for each group of practitioners regulated under a single umbrella Act. The scopes of practice of regulated practitioners specify a number of 'controlled' acts (diagnosis, investigation, prescribing, surgical intervention, and so on) which in turn determines the competencies which regulated practitioners must acquire as part of their training. When calls to regulate a new occupational group arise, the question of whether they should be regulated involves not only an examination of their level of professional organisation and willingness to be regulated, but also of whether they undertake regulated acts. This system of regulation is potentially open to any group of practitioners who undertake the acts regulated by statute. Given that all healthcare practitioners, including CAM and folk healers, 'diagnose' and 'investigate', and some 'prescribe', there would be an argument for including them under such a statutory scheme.

The attraction of this model, or a model like it, is that it could, hypothetically, be applied to all who hold themselves out as healers, limiting their professional activity to diagnosis if need be. It would offer a high level of public protection (by virtue of a register of practitioners, code of ethics, fitness to practise system and so on), and also increase consumer choice by opening up previously restricted practices such as prescribing (previously the exclusive preserve, for example, of the medical profession) to any professional group which has the training and competence to perform that act.

In Ontario, this model accommodates a number of CAM therapies. In Britain's different political climate it may come to be seen as the best model for regulating 'professionalised' CAM therapies, providing a greater level of public protection than would a federal voluntary self-regulating system. But could such a model reasonably accommodate folk healers? Once again, this is related to the professionalism agenda, to the extent that one way of defining professionals is by looking at the characteristics they possess, and in particular their acquisition and possession of 'expert professional knowledge'. Part of the difficulty here is the lack of distinctiveness of folk healers' skills and competencies. Skills held by folk healers may or may not constitute 'professional knowledge', since they are often skills shared by members of a broader, 'lay' population. This makes it hard to determine who should be regulated, and who should not. Because regulation has burdens on registrants, as well as benefits (including, but not limited to, the need to pay subscription fees to a regulatory body, the need to carry insurance, and being subject to a disciplinary regime), it is not generally felt appropriate to extend regulation where it is not required. To give a slightly exaggerated example, no one would reasonably suggest that a mother who rubs a sore child's knee better after a fall needs to be regulated as a therapeutic-touch practitioner. Similarly, much of what is embraced within the notion of healing is not an expert activity (such as massage), even though certain people within a given community may have more aptitude towards it than others.

Measurability and Regulation

The above argument relies on an assumption that in order to regulate a phenomenon, you have to be able to measure it. Certainly, the regulation of medicinal products requires standardisation, with a complex system of clinical trials designed to ensure that a medicine literally does what is says on the box. Evidence-based practice seeks to introduce that same level of standardisation and reproducibility onto the work of healthcare professionals, so that treatments have consistent results irrespective of who provides them. However, the individualised nature of folk healing relies significantly on non-specific effects, whereby much of the therapeutic benefit is derived from the therapeutic relationship itself, including any placebo effects. This focus, together with attention to spiritual, as well as physical and emotional, needs makes it hard to accommodate folk healing within statute or common law. Holistic dimensions of the therapeutic relationship are less amenable to measurement and scientific evaluation. Whilst this fact dominates debates about efficacy and effectiveness, it also has implications for regulation. The determination, for example, of whether a practitioner's fitness to practise is impaired relies explicitly on the ability of a panel to assess a practitioner's acts or omissions against standardised, objective norms. If these do not exist, it is hard to say whether a practitioner did or did not act appropriately in the circumstances.

Implicit in the measurability argument is the idea that the belief, hope and expectation placed in folk healing may be more spiritual than physical in nature, and more akin to religion than healing. Invoking the support of a folk healer to deal with a psychosocial or spiritual malaise may be no more open to regulation than the pursuit of spiritual guidance from a religious minister. This argument has a lot of potency. Acknowledging that CAM has replaced much of what was previously considered 'folk medicine', Stone and Katz note: 'Folk medicine provides mechanisms for coping with ill health as part of the wider context of dealing with misfortune and anxiety. In doing so, it overlaps significantly with cultural and religious beliefs held by the society in which it operates' (Stone and Katz 2005: 159).

Folk Healing, Courts of Law, and Standard of Proof

If there are difficulties in imposing statutory regulation on the activities of folk healers, might regulation by means of common law be an alternative? In short, can folk healers be sued for what they do? The answer is almost certainly not. The difficulties highlighted in relation to measurability may also frustrate the operation of conventional statutory regulation and the common law (Stone and Matthews 1996). From a common law point of view, it is the very lack of evidence as to folk healing's effectiveness that would make it hard to sue a folk healer in a court of law. If it cannot be established that the healing endeavour in question has any efficacy, it would be hard to establish that the intervention caused harm, which is necessary to establish a successful action in negligence or contract. Even though the standard of proof in civil law requires a complainant to demonstrate that it is more likely than not that the harm resulted from the healer's actions, this may prove to be an insurmountable hurdle if 'scientific' evidence can be adduced that the intervention was useless from a therapeutic point of view.

A weakness in the above argument is that it overlooks the need to regulate therapists as well as the healing or purported healing interventions being offered. A central role of formal regulation is to assess suitability for registration of a practitioner, with reference to whether they are a person of 'good health and character'. This is extremely important, although deciding what constitutes either in the case of a folk healer is fraught with difficulty and subjective interpretation.

Nonetheless, a key reason to propose more formalised regulation of folk healers has less to do with the harm they can cause by virtue of the healing services they offer, and more to do with the risks inherent in all therapeutic relationships. These involve abuse of trust and abuse of power, and the literature shows that such abuses occur across all healthcare professions (Halter, Brown and Stone 2007). Folk healers and CAM practitioners can, and do, commit crimes against patients. A folk healer who, for the sake of argument, acts in a sexually inappropriate way, in the guise of treatment or otherwise, would and clearly should be answerable for this unethical and unlawful conduct in a court of law. Whether a patient would feel able to institute a complaint or prosecution is another matter. But it begs the question of whether some level of protection needs to be put in place to ensure that patients are protected from predatory individuals – for example, by way of a criminal records check, or an enquiry into whether or not that person has 'legitimate' therapeutic skills.

Formal Regulatory Approaches Will Not Work

This formulation of the anti-regulation position takes a slightly different view, that even if regulation were imposed, it wouldn't be effective, and that forcing holistic medicine into an incompatible regulatory mould would result either in laws which don't work or in regulation which would strip holistic therapies of their full potential (Stone and Matthews 1996).

This chapter has highlighted some of the ways in which formal regulation is incompatible with folk healing. Many folk healers are not formally educated and trained – another key characteristic of professional practice. They prize their individualism and may actively resist the mantle of professionalism, preferring to see their knowledge as something to be shared and used to empower others. A number of practical difficulties exist. These include: deciding which folk healing practices should be subject to formal regulation; encouraging healers who are not professionally organised to join a single professional register; designing and enforcing a code of ethics covering the diverse beliefs and value systems underpinning the plurality of folk healing practices; populating and implementing any meaningful system of fitness to practise (including the imposition of sanctions) against folk healers whose fitness to practise (health, conduct, or performance) is deemed impaired.

Another pragmatic question concerns whether people would complain about a folk healer to any formal regulatory body were one to exist. This is highly unlikely. The barriers to complaining against CAM practitioners include: the difficulty of judging a highly individualised treatment or service against broadly acceptable professional norms, where none exist; the unwillingness of a complainant to make a complaint against an individual who might be well known and respected in the community, or someone with whom they have a 'dual relationship' (such as neighbour or friend); and finally, the lack of professional indemnity available to therapists offering services which are not professionally organised, so that suing or other attempts to seek financial compensation would probably fail. In the case of folk healers, additional barriers may exist. These are set out in Table 10.2, below.

Table 10.2: Barriers to Bringing a Complaint Against a Folk Healer.

- The recipient's level of expectation as to whether the cure/charm will work
- Attribution of other factors to non-success if it fails (including self-blame and or blame on the part of the healer that the person didn't use the charm properly, or do other things they had been instructed to do
- The fact that the recipient of services may not have paid money for the healing exchange (even though tortuous obligations arise in law whether or not payment is required or given)
- A desire to settle things locally, drawing on other members of the community for informal resolution, including religious or other cultural mechanisms for dealing with sharp practice
- Reliance on the increased role of reputation, and the capacity of an aggrieved person to make their dissatisfaction known in the community, obviating the need or desire for formal regulatory mechanisms

A New Approach to Regulation

This chapter has shown that the current unregulated status of folk healers sits ill with the highly regulated status of conventional health care practitioners and the increasingly regulated status of CAM therapists. Arguments for and against the sustainability of this position have been explored. To the extent that folk healers are offering services routinely understood by the public to be part of CAM, it seems that folk healers could similarly be encouraged to pursue voluntary forms of regulation, to help to ensure that they are practising within broad professional norms as these begin to emerge. That said, real problems have been identified in imposing formal regulation, be it voluntary or statutory, across the diverse and fragmented realm of folk healing.

Nonetheless, it would be erroneous to think that the only model of regulation that could be applied to folk healers is that which currently applies to conventional healthcare practitioners, CAM therapists and other (non healthcare) professionals. Freedom to practise needs to be tempered by the need to protect patients who may be vulnerable from exploitation. Research is needed to explore the feasibility of alternative forms of regulation, such as licensing folk healers. A licensing system would not depend on the purported efficacy of the practice offered, but could ensure, for example, that criminal records checks have been carried out, indemnity cover is held, and that any premises which services are offered from are safe and insured. This compromise situation may not provide the full range of protection that is in place for other healthcare professionals, but it could prove to be a proportionate regulatory response, especially given the difficulties in applying other models of regulation.

Without wishing to restrict unduly the range of therapists offering services, or the services which they offer, realistic and achievable restrictions should be placed on folk healers which strike an appropriate balance between recognising the freedom of individuals to choose services whilst providing a level of protection expected in any other service industry. Most folk healers operate, hopefully, with high levels of healing intent and act fully in accordance with the ethical and societal expectations placed upon them. But some level of external intervention may be required to provide patients with the reassurance that their hopes, trust and expectations are at the very least being placed in someone whose good faith, if not skills, can be relied upon.

Notes

1. Herbal medicine has been regulated for centuries, the earliest formal recognition being found in the so-called 'Quacks' Charter of 1542, which legalised lay herbalism, provided the services of herbalists were offered for free. Currently, Section 12(1) of the UK Medicines Act 1968 specifies an exemption for herbal medicines from licensing provided that they are supplied subsequent to a one-to-one consultation. Section 12(2) exempts herbal medicines provided that they are produced according to standard traditional, non-industrial methods. Herbal remedies now fall under EU legislation and need to be registered as part of the Traditional Herbal Medicines Registration Scheme required by Directive 2004/24/EC, which came into effect on 30 October 2005. See: http://www.ehpa.eu/medicines_legislation/index.html.
2. The government's White Paper (DoH 2007) sets out a vision for the future regulation of statutorily regulated health professionals in the U.K. The policies contained in this document represent a culmination of five years work following the Shipman Inquiry Report, by Dame Janet Smith, who reviewed regulation in the wake of the U.K.'s biggest health scandal: the murder by Harold Shipman, a general practitioner, of some 250 of his patients, and set out proposals for reform in her fifth report. See Smith, J. (2004). Shipman Fifth Report - Safeguarding Patients: Lessons from the Past - Proposals for the Future. Command Paper Cm 6394. http://www.the-shipman-inquiry.org.uk/fifthreport.asp (accessed 3 September 2009).
3. The U.K. Department of Health continues to consider moving acupuncture, herbal medicine and traditional Chinese medicine (TCM) towards statutory regulation under the auspices of the Health Professions Council. Failure to achieve statutory regulation may prohibit herbal medicine practitioners from prescribing herbal medicines in the future. Department of Health (2009) http://www.dh.gov.uk/en/Consultations/Liveconsultations/DH_103567 (accessed 3 September 2009). Funding from the Department of Health to the Prince of Wales's Foundation for Integrated Health led, in 2008, to the creation of the Complementary and Natural Healthcare Council, creating a federal system of voluntary self-regulation (see: http://www.cnhc.org.uk/pages/index.cfm – accessed 3 September 2009). Moves to bring a number of CAM therapies under a federal system of voluntary regulation have concentrated, in the first instance, on eleven highly professionalised CAM therapies.

4. Because untrained and unsupervised practitioners can cause considerable harm to patients in an unregulated environment, market forces, which operate retrospectively, provide an inadequate level of public protection. For further discussion, see Stone and Matthews (1996).
5. Under the Osteopaths Act 1993 and Chiropractors Act 1994 respectively.
6. The wording of these statutes will probably be changed as part of the current White Paper reforms in Britain of regulation, shifting the role of promotion, more appropriately, to professional associations.
7. See HM Treasury (2005).
8. The adoption of this approach has been seen as somewhat contrary to the underlying purpose of healthcare (as distinct from business) regulation – namely, patient protection.
9. Thus, in the statutory sector, the General Dental Council now regulates dental technicians and hygienists, as well as dentists; the Nursing and Midwifery Council regulates nurses, midwives and specialist community public health nurses; and the Health Professions Council regulates thirteen separate therapies (arts practitioners, biomedical scientists, chiropodists and podiatrists, clinical scientists, dieticians, occupational practitioners, operating department practitioners, orthoptists, paramedics, physiotherapists, prosthetists and orthotists, radiographers and speech and language practitioners), and is soon to regulate applied psychologists, counselling and psychotherapy as well as the CAM therapies discussed.
10. Not only does TM account for the majority of primary healthcare in Africa, in Asia and Latin America populations continue to use TM as a result of historical circumstances and cultural beliefs. In China, TM accounts for around 40 per cent of all healthcare delivered. The WHO report additionally notes that TM providers include both TM practitioners and allopathic medicine professionals such as doctors, dentists and nurses who provide TM/CAM therapies to their patients – e.g., many medical doctors also use acupuncture to treat their patients.
11. A simplified licensing scheme for traditional herbal medicinal products, administered in the U.K. by the Medicines and Healthcare Products Regulatory Agency (MHRA), was introduced as a result of the Traditional Herbal Medicinal Products Directive (2004/24/EC).
12. Article 2 of EC Regulation 172/2002 defines food or foodstuff as 'any substance or product, whether processed, partially processed or unprocessed, intended to be, or reasonably expected to be ingested by humans'.
13. The tort (civil wrong) of negligence arises when a person has a duty of care, acts in breach of care, and by dint of action or failure to act causes someone harm. Where the offer to treat and the acceptance of that offer is the

subject of a legally binding agreement (a contract), an almost identical action arises in the form of an action for breach of contract.

14. One can argue that consumers should be free to make choices, but still argue that all people holding themselves out as therapists should be regulated.
15. Calls for greater transparency and openness of this type of regulation underpin the White Paper's attempts to increase consumer involvement and participation, and counterbalance professional control with a broader stakeholder base; hence, a new term of art emerging: stakeholder regulation (see DoH 2007).
16. For a discussion of how Ontario's Health Professions Act, 1991 (RHPA) operates, see HPRAC (2001).

References

DoH. 2007. 'Trust, Assurance and Safety: The Regulation of Health Professionals in the Twenty-first Century', Cm 7013. London: HMSO.

Eskinazi, D. 1998. 'Factors that Shape Alternative Medicine', *Journal of the American Medical Association* 280(18): 1621–1623.

Halter, M., H. Brown and J. Stone. 2007. *Sexual Boundary Violations By Health Employees: An Overview Of The Published Empirical Literature*. Council For Healthcare Regulatory Excellence, London.

HM Treasury. 2005. 'Reducing Administrative Burdens: Effective Inspection And Enforcement', report of the Hampton Review. Retrieved 3 September 2009 from http://www.berr.gov.uk/files/file22988.pdf.

House of Lords. 2000. 'Complementary and Alternative Medicine', report of the Select Committee on Science and Technology, HL Paper 123. London: HMSO.

HPRAC. 2001. 'Adjusting The Balance: A Review of the Regulated Health Professions Act'. Ontario: Health Professions Regulatory Advisory Council.

Jack, P. 2006. 'Exploring a Federal Approach to Voluntary Self-regulation of Complementary Healthcare: A Consultation Document'. London: Prince of Wales's Foundation For Integrated Health.

National Working Group. 2005. 'Report of The National Working Group on the Regulation of Complementary Therapists to the Minister for Health and Children'. Dublin: The Stationery Office.

Shipman Inquiry (2004). 'Safeguarding Patients: Lessons From The Patient, Proposals For The Future', 5th Report. Cm 6394. Retrieved 3 September 2009 from: http://www.the-shipman-inquiry.org.uk/reports.asp.

Stone, J. 2005a. 'Development Of Proposals For A Future Voluntary Regulatory Structure For Complementary Health Care Professions' report commissioned by the Prince Of Wales's Foundation For Integrated Health. London: Prince Of Wales's Foundation For Integrated Health.

———. 2005b. 'Regulation of CAM Practitioners: Reflecting on the Last Ten Years', *Complementary Therapies In Clinical* Practice 11(1): 5–10.

Stone, J. and J. Katz. 2005. 'Understanding Health And Healing', in T. Heller, G. Lee-Treweek, J. Katz, J. Stone and S. Spurr (eds), *Perspectives on Complementary and Alternative Medicine*. London: Routledge.

Stone, J. and J. Matthews. 1996. *Complementary Medicine and the Law*. Oxford: Oxford University Press.

Vickers, A. and T. Heller. 2005. 'Traditional, Folk and Cultural Perspectives of CAM', in T. Heller, G. Lee-Treweek, J. Katz, J. Stone and S. Spurr (eds), *Perspectives on Complementary and Alternative Medicine*. London: Routledge.

Walshe, K. and L. Benson. 2005. 'Time For Radical Reform', *British Medical Journal* 330(7506): 1504–1506.

WHO 2000. General Guidelines for Methodologies on Research and Evaluation of Traditional Medicine. World Health Organization, Geneva. WHO/EDM/TRM/2000.http://whqlibdoc.who.int/hq/2000/WHO_EDM_TRM_2000.1.pdf (accessed 3 September 2009).

WHO 2002. 'WHO Strategy For Traditional Medicine, 2002–2005'. Geneva: World Health Organisation.

WHO 2003. 'Traditional Medicine Factsheet'. Retrieved 3 September 2009 from: http://www.who.int/mediacentre/factsheets/fs134/en/.

Chapter 11

Epilogue: Towards Authentic Medicine: Bodies and Boundaries

Stuart McClean and Ronnie Moore

In Britain and Ireland, as elsewhere in the Western world, our appetite for texts, research, policy and public debate in the field of complementary and alternative medicine (CAM) shows no sign of abating, and yet much of this activity has largely neglected the sub-field of folk healing and medicine. Folk healing still remains relegated to the status of either 'traditional' medicine, with spurious connotations of prerational and premodern thinking, or ethnomedicine, again with its own set of essentialist assumptions about regional ethnic 'traditions'. The chapters that make up this volume highlight a rapidly changing picture. They have mapped out the diversity of folk healing in modern Britain and Ireland, as well as pointing towards the sheer complexity, contestability and fluidity of the boundaries between heterodox folk and CAM practices, as well as biomedicine(s).

These chapters form a series of answers to a previous set of questions about the nature and role of folk-healing practices within the available panoply of CAM in contemporary Britain and Ireland. In the spirit of inquiry, this volume has also raised new questions about the nature of healing, health beliefs and the boundaries of healing knowledge. The chapters all address the complexity of these issues as well as the nature of healing plurality. The volume also offers a call for more empirical work into the diversity as well as the commonalities of all medical and healing practices in Western societies – the shared symbolic and metaphorical nature of sickness and healing (over and above the physical and physiological). Within this schema, biomedicine, CAM, folk medicine and other orthodox and heterodox health practices are placed loosely within a cultural 'system', each interdependent and interacting with the other in a continuing spiral of meaning and signification.

Within the wider cultural sphere or system, folk-healing practices operate in tandem with scientific formal biomedicine, and as such the majority of chapters in this volume enter into simultaneous dialogue about the nature of formal medicine and its role in helping us to place and understand the nature of folk healing. Folk-healing ideology and practices primarily operate outside formal medical ideology, and yet these practices hold a particular relationship and association with science and rationalism: '[folk healing supports] a shared experience of disease within the community outside of school medicine, or Western scientific medicine ... [folk healing] involves rational and irrational elements; empirical and magical elements' (Vaskilampi 1981: 3). Vaskilampi's statement indicates that folk healing is much more nuanced than has been hitherto suggested. The continued existence of folk healing and its current revival, revitalisation and reinvention suggest that it is not the handmaiden of formal medicine, its existence is not provisional or contingent on the continued good will of medical science: 'Folk medicine does not exist at the mercy of bio-medicine!' (Alver 1995: 30).

In the U.S. it has been shown that folk medicine practices are confined to the poor and the uneducated (Blaustein 1992); and yet, CAM practices are perceived to be predominantly the preserve of the wealthy and consumer-oriented middle classes (Sharma 1995). We would suggest that both assumptions are erroneous and only serve to simplify taxonomic differences between CAM and folk healing, although the question of cost and affordability for non-orthodox healing is also crucial and cannot be put aside. The reasons why people use folk healing in Britain and Ireland today, amongst the plethora of available treatments and cures, should no longer be surprising. Sickness, particularly that which is threatening to the self and the body, brings to the fore considerations about 'cultural' responses to sickness: 'In sickness, more so than any other vicissitude of life, people will throw caution to the wind, as it were, and resort to trials and actions that they might not consider under ordinary circumstances' (Hand 1980: xxv). Ongoing debate surrounding 'biographical disruption' (the impact of ill health on normalised constructions of identity and the life course) has thrown additional light on this salient theme (see Bury 1982; Becker 1997). Folk healing, then, provides a range of non-specific benefits, a source of control over hopeless situations, a form of power and knowledge that confers 'expert' status on its participants. Its attractiveness therefore 'serves a number of psychosocial functions not met exclusively by scientific medicine' (Mathews 1987: 889).

Our debate about the nature of the boundaries between folk, CAM and formal medicine resonate with Kleinman's seminal analysis of the health care system as 'a local cultural system composed of three overlapping parts: the popular, professional and folk sectors' (Kleinman 1980: 50). Kleinman's original model suggested that the popular sector referred to the lay, culturally specific treatment of sickness; the professional sector denoted organised healing professions; and the folk sector captured the specialist, non-professional sector encompassing secular and sacred healers. This book largely confirms the significance of Kleinman's model, but suggests that the ways in which the boundaries between folk, professional and lay sectors overlap are significant and surprising. For example, in MacFarlane and de Brún's (Chapter 8, this volume) analysis we see how migrants' perceptions of biomedicine(s) are influenced by folk and culturally contingent health beliefs.

Folk Healing, Globalisation and 'Community' Engagement

In the WHO's 'Traditional Medicine Strategy, 2002–2005' (WHO 2002), the role of 'traditional medicine' in a global context is highlighted, emphasising that in many 'developing' countries traditional medicine is clearly more widely available than allopathic Western medicine, a situation that is particularly true of rural areas. The document's authors recognise that traditional medicine is 'often embedded in wider belief systems and continues to be an integral and important part of many people's lives' (ibid.: 13), whereas in 'developed' countries the situation differs significantly in that people are more critical of their use of biomedicine, hence a greater reliance on complementary approaches.

In considering the global influence of CAM and traditional medicine, the WHO point to four key areas that pose the greatest challenge to its future: national policy and regulatory frameworks; safety, efficacy and quality; access; and rational use. Each area points to a stumbling block to CAM and traditional medicine's wider use and acceptance, and it appears optimistic at the level at which CAM and traditional medicine can become integrated with formal medicine. However, the chapters in this volume highlight the importance and relevance of, as well as the reliance on, 'folk' medicine (broadly understood) in Western societies. The situations and contexts highlighted here are not necessarily comparable with the traditional medicine that the WHO alludes to. As Stone suggests (Chapter 10, this volume), the view of the WHO on traditional medicine is different when it comes to folk healing. In many societies, folk treatments are more likely to be considered mainstream treatments and can therefore fit under a regulatory remit in a way that many individualistic, ad hoc folk treatments in the West cannot.

Moreover, Chinese and Ayurvedic medicine are important reminders of complete, holistic and alternative health belief systems and practices. In addition, whole systems have been ignored because they were exotic, or foreign to the sensitivities of the Western European imagination, as well as those that did not proliferate or dominate or were lost in history. The Mongol hordes, for example, were reputed to have ransacked and destroyed libraries and medical information in their wake.

In recent years globalisation has captured the attention of political and social scientists, economists and others (Held et al. 1999). Globalisation involves increasing local, cultural, national, international and intercontinental migration, social networking, interaction and exchange. In addition, globalisation has delivered traditional beliefs and practices from multiple world cultures to the door of the Western surgery and to the hospital. It also infers that formal medicine will find it increasingly difficult to ignore alternative medical beliefs and practices. Such processes of inward migration and cross-cultural reference in the West have equally helped question the so-called standardised science and pre-eminence of biomedicine; the monopoly is now being seriously challenged. And a looming crisis in biomedicine might suggest that we are on the cusp of a new paradigm as medical boundaries undergo further 'blurring'.

In response to the House of Lords (2000) report, there have been serious attempts to introduce and integrate complementary medicine with front line medical services, albeit on a short-term-trial basis only. Several independent audits have now been produced (for example, for Haringey and South Islington in London), and these have indicated that illness severity has been reduced, quality of life improved, and doctors are referring patients to these services (Peters, Andrews and Hills 2006; Robinson 2006). These trials were extended and introduced to two health centres in Northern Ireland in 2007/8.

Despite being a collection about Britain and Ireland, we do not hold to traditional anthropological notions about the significance of place and the localisation of the object of study,[1] hence the notable absence of Scotland from our empirical studies. Chapters such as Philpin's (Chapter 4) analysis of wool measuring practices in Wales seem to be the exception in that the 'rootedness' of folk healing is seen as a consequence of the 'ordinariness' and mundanity of healing (see also Chapter 5, this volume); other chapters problematise localisation given the widespread effects of migration and globalisation (Chapter 8) and of social transformations on the nature of folk and alternative health knowledge (Chapters 6 and 7).

Nevertheless, the rootedness of folk healing in particular contexts and communities, however broadly defined, may give us some additional clues as to its importance and its resistance to formal regulatory structures, in the form of licensing, for example. Sitting as it does outside formal regulatory structures (see Chapter 10, this volume), folk healing relies on its ties to community-held, lay conceptualisations of health and sickness, cultural beliefs and wider accounts of health. Such beliefs often overlap with religious, or more broadly spiritual, beliefs, hence it is perhaps no surprise that during the nineteenth century the true rival to the folk healer was the clergy, and not, as previously suspected, the physician.

The essence of the folk healer is less to do with expert knowledge and more to do with needs mediated through the type of solidarity that Durkheim described.[2] Through the collective representations of society, we reason that it is in our interests to obey (Hamilton 2001: 113). Here the expert witness resting on the defence of individual culpability may be seriously challenged. The debates are not new, but have been played out in other places and in other periods, notably by Diderot, Hobbes and Hume. Culpability relates to free will, but this may be a 'theoretical liberty'. Durkheim, for example, emphatically pursues the power of the social, and the view that people are not only individual agents.

The social is important for many communities, and the healer fulfils a role based on community expectation and community obligation; unlike the CAM healer, the folk healer has not necessarily chosen a career but has been thrown into a role (and its attendant expectations) conferred by birthright, talent and so on. As Lee-Treweek states (Chapter 9, this volume), healers address needs 'deep in the heart of their locales', reinforcing the sense that folk healing is most suited to serving the psychosocial needs of the local community.

For the CAM therapist, the issue of culpability is more straightforward in that the CAM healer represents and is the embodiment of particular, albeit specialised, professional standards conferred by training and practice. Thus, CAM has unwittingly bought into the biomedical paradigm on issues connected with risk and public safety. Stone's highly significant discussion of legal issues concerning culpability therefore become more complex when one considers the healer as not acting alone and narcissistically in accordance with some modernist notions of 'professional role', but acting with the full influence, support and weight of expectation within the community. Prevailing debates, led by both the Department of Health and the WHO, amongst others, about licensing, regulation and safety, are problematic and miss the point in the case of folk healing because of the lay-inspired nature of the folk healer's work, beliefs and role.

As commercially oriented healthcare systems, biomedicine and, increasingly CAM, are bound up with professionalisation and commoditisation: socio-economic processes that folk healing has, to date, significantly resisted. Indeed, commoditisation is something of a hallmark of more professionalised forms of CAM, where entrepreneurialism largely dominates as business practice (see Chapter 7, 9, and 10, this volume). In contrast, folk healing has, historically, had more of a resistance to professionalising, and an antipathy to money (or sometimes an ambivalence to standardised monetary forms of exchange). In Chapters 3, 4, 5, 7 and 9, this volume, for example, healers show a dislike for or shun payment with money, preferring instead to work for free or to take payment in kind for their services, which, we should remind ourselves, is seen in the context of community 'resource' or capital. As Stone explains by way of definition (Chapter 10, this volume), folk healing has 'remained outside economically defined and commercially oriented healthcare systems, and has, to date, significantly resisted commoditization'.

In some ways a discussion of money can lead us into a useful typology about the range of CAM and folk healing practice and, indeed the reasons behind the blurring of the boundaries between them (as suggested in Chapter 7, this volume). From Simmel we inherited the notion that money was a doubled-edge sword: it liberated people from age-old status ties and distinctions but at the same time it transformed societies from *gemeinschaft* (organic community) to *Gesellschaft* (the instrumentalism of modern society) (Simmel 1990 [1907]). Although an instrument and symbol of freedom, money also represented one of the de-personalising features of modernity, and was thus seen by many anthropologists and social scientists as an evil – the money as 'acid' hypothesis (Maurer 2006). Bloch and Parry also voiced such sentiments in their seminal anthology on money, morality and exchange: 'Destructive of community, money depersonalises social relations' (1989: 6).

In many folk healing transactions money is not perceived as an appropriate form of exchange for healing services, but then the same is true for some healing services within CAM, where entrepreneurial healers allow for some variation (as well as pragmatism) in the monetary repertoires that ordinary people adopt in their everyday lives. Such non-monetarised relationships are not as unusual as one might at first assume from traditional economic analyses of Western societies, and can be further illustrated in the widespread practice of such diverse activities as baby-sitting exchanges, car pools, etc (see Melitz 1970). As an impersonal system of commodity exchange we can see how the exchange of money may seem inappropriate in some healing transactions, particularly more so where those relationships are bounded within the personal ties of the local community; here, money exchange may be awkward or suggestive of different kinds of 'professional' relationship not warranted by the therapeutic encounter: 'There is therefore something profoundly awkward about offering it as a gift expressive of relationships which are supposed to be personal, enduring, moral and altruistic' (Bloch and Parry 1989: 9).

Science, Scientism and Faith: Paradigms, Tensions and Pragmatism

Historically, the medical establishment has acknowledged the persistent presence of what it has described as 'alternative health practices' in Western societies, but it has in general ignored and/or belittled traditional ideas surrounding magic, superstition, religion and, consequently, health and illness. In addition, the teaching of formal medicine remains conservative and largely devoid of an emic perspective; and yet, the empirical evidence presented here suggests that the relationship between formal medicine and folk medicine is highly complex and involves a degree of dependency. The public face of formal biomedicine remains largely paternalistic and antagonistic to folk medicine, not to mention CAM practices. Yet modern medicine reframes 'magical' practice as placebos, and there is much in modern medicine that is not fully scientifically understood. Innovative new therapies, for example, have been shown to be effective and are now routinely deployed in front-line services in psychiatric and clinical psychological practices. For example, Eye Movement Desensitization and Reprocessing (EMDR), involving rapid sensory movement from side to side (visual or audible), appears to enable patients to deal with traumatic events (Shapiro 2001; Shapiro and Forrest 2004).

A central question remains: How do heathcare systems earn and retain credibility? Historians have illustrated a redrawing of conceptual boundaries. Distinctions between magical practices, religion and science are fluid and contingent. Medicine is often taken as a metaphor for religion and the parallels are stark. Trevor-Roper's detailed work on the interconnectedness of the histories of religion and medicine in the sixteenth and seventeenth centuries is illustrative of this (Trevor-Roper 2006).

Religions offer a guide for living and are concerned with saving mortal souls, with the promise of life after death, but the demise of religion and the rise of an atheist ideology may mean the disintegration of rules, laws and moral obligations in a way that would be unimaginable and at worst be tantamount to societal collapse in a manner described by Diamond (2005). The crises in the established Church may be mirrored by a looming crisis in Western medicine if formal medicine continues to maintain a status quo position in regard to the outright dismissal of alternative health and medical practices. The central point to emphasise here is that multiple health beliefs and systems have always existed and continue to exist in Britain and Ireland.

If we accept Cox's (Chapter 3, this volume) analysis of medicine's attitude towards folk healing in nineteenth-century Ireland, then we can see that folk healing was not faced with complete antagonism; rather, orthodox accounts and endorsements of folk treatments were accompanied by a scientism that was intrinsic to that particular way of thinking; that is, a gloss of scientific-sounding language was often used to explain how folk cures and potions worked. Today, this scientism is prevalent not only in the wider response to CAM and heterodox treatments – for example, through requesting inappropriate clinical trials of treatments and so on, emphasising scientism's exclusionary and elitist nature – but also in CAM practitioners' ever-changing discourse of healing: scientific-sounding language is increasingly used in the justification of such treatments, and mimicry of perceived biomedical treatments has permeated the discourse and practice of even the most esoteric of healing practices (McClean 2003). Folk healing is not outside the scope of scientific enquiry but it is clear to us that its voice and authority should be heard as one amongst the panoply of available voices and discourses; equally, scientific knowledge and its attendant ontological and epistemological assumptions and dogma are not beyond public scrutiny (Habermas 1971).

Folk and indigenous medicines predate the dominant and highly professionalised formal system of biomedicine. Biomedicine, however, whether it approves or not, is now in a position where it is repeatedly being forced to recognise alternative forms of medical and healthcare practice (the increase in medical articles in both the popular and academic press indicate a recognition that they must respond to a perceived crisis). There are a number of reasons for this. Firstly, formal medicine has lost sight of its main function. The key objective is the health of the individual (and communities). The rush for scientific discovery has meant that biomedicine has veered away from a holistic understanding of medical conditions (considered crucially important for well-being by early Greek and other physicians, such as Hippocrates) and followed a specific scientifically driven path. Even Galen believed that authoritative learning should not be followed blindly. And while the scope of medicine has expanded to include a wide variety of paramedical, pharmaceutical and associated industries, its focus has progressively narrowed. The seriousness of this is repeatedly reflected in the annual proceedings of national and international medical sociological conferences, where research papers on the physician–patient relationship have come to be expected.

Secondly, formal medicine has also been attacked for breaking its own basic principles – such as 'first do no harm'. The sociological literature is replete with examples of the iatrogenic consequences of formal medicine (see Szasz 1961; Illich 1976; Navarro 1986), and there are other medical concerns, ranging from the well-documented thalidomide cases to recent drug-testing disasters that have killed and incapacitated volunteers, as well as organ theft and surgery for convenience. We may add to this the unashamed rise in medicine as a body and/or gender-enhancement industry, offering popular Western media-driven idealised versions of body image, ranging from pursuing the Adonis or 'six pack' complex to size zero. This often involves dangerous procedures – such as taking drugs to increase muscle size, or using botulinum toxin (botox), an extremely poisonous natural substance, or undergoing major 'cosmetic' surgery to enhance or reduce the size of various parts of the body. The physical and psychological affects of these services and their procedures are now attracting significant debate (Bordo 1998; Sullivan 2001).[3]

In addition, modern pressures in medicine have also had an impact on medical practitioners themselves, with some possibly having lost their way and experiencing a sense of anomie. While we may not hear about the extent of such anomie, we may take as a marker certain signposts, as with the extreme cases of Dr Harold Shipman and Dr Neary.[4] We may add to this other notable scandals, such as blood contamination (see Barrett, Moore and Staines 2007).

In recent years, anthropologists and sociologists have looked at the relationship between medicine, modernity and risk (Douglas 1975; Beck 1992; Luhmann 1993), as well as trust (Sztompka 1999). Douglas argues that the institutions of the society in which we live frame our perceptions of risk. When a physical disaster occurs it is keenly studied and the performance of community institutions is assessed. Blame comes to fall in such a way as to reinforce the local community ideal. Questions of risk and blame reach individuals in terms of a choice to be made whether to reinforce the authority of institutions or subvert them (Douglas 1992). While modernity has reduced some risk it also introduced new forms hitherto unknown, and therefore with new conditions come new risks; individuals and institutions need to be reflexive in order to modify their knowledge and to nullify risk. Late modernity is characterised by anxiety and organised reaction to it. Biomedicine, which promised so much, has become defensive in the face of increasing lawsuits for malpractice.

As in previous chapters, our analysis of formal medicine and modernity has suggested that its emphasis on objective truth should be set against a more multifaceted conception of 'truth' closer to that of the arts and humanities (see Vattimo 1991; Zabala 2006). In particular, the contemporary Italian philosopher Gianni Vattimo (1991), a close adherent of the American philosopher Richard Rorty, provides a way through the debate about postmodernity and the nature of knowledge systems. In line with other postmodern critics, such as Jean-Francois Lyotard and Zygmunt Bauman, Vattimo suggests that we are currently experiencing a deep pluralism in Western societies brought about by a proliferation of multiple points of view; a rejection and replacement of the Western 'unitary' version of history. Whereas in previous historical circumstances under conditions of modernity one particular hegemonic world-view (such as the scientific one) would gain sway, under postmodern conditions the markers of legitimacy become equally proliferated, and hence more and more individuals, representing multiple discourses, are able to have their say. For Vattimo such a proliferation of discourses and points of view (as well as 'truths') is exacerbated by the role of the mass media and mass communications, the result of a society of 'generalised communication'. Our story of folk healing appears therefore to be one of multiple and competing stories: the 'eclipse' of folk medicine; the rise to prominence and hegemony of biomedicine; the crisis of contemporary health care systems; the New Age and ushering in of a new consciousness; the individual narratives of healers and their patients; and the computerisation and democratisation of health knowledge.

However, set against Vattimo's extreme relativist position, the British philospher Roy Bhaskar recognises that witnessed 'truths' may only be part of the story. Bhaskar recognises that social structures are different from natural structures because the former are both produced by social activity and reproduce that activity (Blaikie 2007: 192). Bhaskar has argued that our knowledge of truth is transient but recognises an intransigent reality that, although it may not be directly witnessed, is known by its effects. Bhaskar therefore attempts to transcend the opposed positions of science and interpretivism, arguing that while our knowledge of the real world is transient, the real world exists independently of our knowledge of it, and reality is intransigent. Theories accounting for reality are not perfect and can change, but the point Bhaskar is making is that if something is shown to exist (by its effects) then it must be real. We might understand this as a pragmatic view of 'truth' (ibid.: 202), and in this sense it is similar to Searle's (1996) defence of realism, contrasting 'brute facts' (those that exist independently of human thoughts) and 'social facts' (those that are observer-relative).

Bhaskar does not believe, as Harre, Vattimo and others do, that it is only social agents and not social structures that make things happen, 'the collective action effect' (Blaikie 2007: 150). He attempts a middle stance between positivism and hermeneutics, science and interpretation (ibid.: 146). These positions have led others to suggest that the story is incomplete if we only focus on 'independent, knowable reality', or if we accept the idea of 'multiple and incommensurate socially constructed realities'. This highlights perceptions of the social world rather than what is real. These are the falsehoods (epistemic shifts or fallacies) underscored by social theorists such as Kuhn and Foucault.

Recent social science offers a new ontology that incorporates system analysis to overcome the limitations of the falsehoods described by Kuhn and others (Cilliers 1998, 2005; Capra 2002, 2005). The 'complexity turn' is illustrative of this. It involves 'the interdisciplinary understanding of reality as composed of complex open systems with emergent properties and transformational potential' (Byrne, cited in Blaikie 2007: 207). It is anti-reductionist and 'is seen as steering a course between modernism and postmodernism by rejecting the former's rigid formalism and determinism and the latter's reaction and irrationalism' (Reed and Harvey, cited in ibid.: 211).

Perceptions of what is real impinge on treatment and care and directly affect the well-being of individuals and communities. The question of what counts as real is therefore of concern. Keith Thomas (1973) attempted to solve the reason for the change in what counted as real and the shift from magic and religion to rationality, but he failed to appreciate the enduring presence of magic and superstition that subliminally and directly influences our lives (whether we adhere to magical belief or not).

The point is not that we have shifted from one paradigm to another as a simple transaction; rather, we move within and between 'magical' and 'scientific' worlds as and when we need to, or when it suits us, and this is context bound. In other words, there are multiple realities (Vattimo 1991), some are interpretive but others are enduring (Bhaskar 1979). Magic and science live together and occupy the same social reality, they collide, collude and are codependent.

For Malinowski and Thomas, magic was a response to difficult and dangerous living experiences. The question is: Why is folk healing important in relatively affluent Western societal contexts? The Enlightenment may have obscured and subverted the real nature of health knowledge and health care. We would argue that the pragmatic use of multiple healthcare systems, according to the ethnographic data presented here, offers a way to overcome the Foucauldian impasse described by Wahlberg (Chapter 6, this volume).

The history of medicine, formal and traditional, suggests a battle for bodies, whereby organised Western biomedicine came to dominate in terms of legitimacy, control and occupational protectionism. Just as religion tended to proselytise, medicine tended to medicalise. The medical profession became adept in dominating the medical labour market, effectively eliminating competition (McQuaide 2005: 287), and the justificatory rhetoric for this was science. Scientific concepts came to replace traditional (quasi-religious) notions of illness. However, secular and scientific medicines did not simply replace folk or lay medical practice. Bakx (1991), for example, shows that such traditional practices did not cease; rather, they survived in even the most politically unsympathetic landscapes, such as the former Soviet Union.

The resurgence in popularity of alternative medical systems is more properly seen as a 'revival' or 'reinvention' rather than a survival. It is now well-acknowledged that the revival and rediscovery of alternative medicine is becoming increasingly popular in the Western world, although biomedicine could arguably be seen to have won the historical struggle for dominance (though this victory is neither complete nor enduring). On the basis of the narratives and observations presented here, it would be wrong to assume that the public and local communities have completely accepted scientific medicine without question. For us, 'authentic medicine'[5] includes folk medicine. Folk healing, therefore, continues to exist and remains an important part of healthcare resources in the West.

As we have suggested, globalisation has made us more cross-culturally aware and in a way that is unprecedented. Instant information means that lay people are Internet savvy or 'Internet positive'. Physicians now ensure they provide verifiable and accurate knowledge; they are also under pressure to offer a service required of them by a better-educated public. So while both informal and alternative medicine are now commercially exploited in the U.S. (McQuaide 2005) and Britain and Ireland (Cant and Sharma, cited in Albrecht, Fitzpatrick and Scrimshaw 2000), an argument against a tendency toward their 'commoditisation' is that it has existed precisely because it could not be bought, codified or regulated. Curers require no payment for what is, in essence, a community resource or cultural capital.

Finally, we accept that in our consideration of folk healing practices in Britain and Ireland we are likely to raise numerous questions as well as controversies, and we are happy if this is the case. What is clear to us is that, as a subject area, this should not be constrained by the limits of a single discipline, and while we recognise that trespassing onto the terrain of other academic disciplines carries risks, it is important to take such risks; indeed, we would actively encourage such interdisciplinary dialogue and fraternity. In addition to anthropology and sociology, clearly history, medicine, psychology, philosophy, theology, folklore and linguistics all have a significant role to play in the debate, and boundaries need to be transgressed to reveal a more complex and nuanced picture of multiple health belief systems and health behaviour than the one we have offered here. Through our empirical and conceptual observations we have merely tried to shine a small light in different directions.

Notes

1. Traditional anthropological studies reflect a past concern with the localisation of the object of study. See Gupta and Ferguson (1997) and Rapport and Dawson (1998) for critiques.
2. Although Durkheim looks specifically at religion, we would argue that the effect is the same.
3. Clinical psychologist Tanya Byron has looked at body image and why individuals cause self-harm to meet social pressures about what is perceived to be normal. She has shown how vulnerable young people risk death and develop real psychiatric problems in pursuit of idealised notions of body image. See Am I Normal? , BBC 1 documentary, 29 April 2008.
4. Dr Harold Shipman was convicted of murdering a large number of his patients. He was himself a recreational drug-taker and began to administer lethal doses of diamorphine to his patients, forging their medical certificates to suggest that they had poor health. Dr Neary was the subject of the the Harding Clark Report (2006), which showed that he performed an inordinate number of unnecessary Caesarean hysterectomies on young women at Our Lady of Lourdes Hospital in Drogheda, Ireland. The report raised questions about paternalistic and arrogant medical culture, medical training and professionalism because doctors' activities were not policed, even by close colleagues. Dr Neary practised until 1998 and was then struck off the medical register. While concerns were raised in the report, and indeed in the recent Madden report on organ retention, it suggested that the maternity unit at Lourdes Hospital (owned until 1997 by the religious order the Medical Missionaries of Mary) appeared to be living in a 'time warp'. The report added that there was almost an 'epidemic' of peripartum hysterectomy there as late as 1996. It also went on to say that Dr Neary's colleagues speak very highly of him and have universally expressed amazement that he was struck off.
5. 'Authentic medicine' refers to that which is recognised as and deemed genuine in that it is believed to affect health.

References

Albrecht A., R. Fitzpatrick and S. Scrimshaw (eds). 2000. *The Handbook of Social Studies in Health and Medicine*. London: Sage.

Alver, B.G. 1995. 'The Bearing of Folk Belief on Cure and Healing', *Journal of Folklore Research* 32(1): 21–33.

Bakx, K. 1991. 'The "Eclipse" of Folk Medicine in Western Society', *Sociology of Health and Illness* 13(1): 20–35.

Bordo, S. 1998. 'Braveheart, Babe, and the Contemporary Body', in E. Parens (ed.) *Enhancing Human Traits: Ethical and Social Implications*. Washington, DC: Georgetown University Press.

Barrett, R., R. Moore and A. Staines. 2007. 'Blood Transfusion in Ireland: Perceptions of Risk, a Question of Trust', *Health, Risk and Society* 9(4): 375–88.

Beck, U. 1992. *Risk Society: Towards a New Modernity*. London: Sage.

Bhaskar, R. 1979. *The Possibility of Naturalism: A Philosophical Critique of the Contemporary Human Sciences*. Brighton: Harvester.

Blaikie, N. 2007. *Approaches to Social Inquiry*, 2nd edn. Cambridge: Polity.

Blaustein, R. 1992. 'Traditional Healing Today: Moving Beyond Stereotypes', in J. Kirkland, H.F. Mathews, C.W. Sullivan and K. Baldwin (eds), *Herbal and Magical Medicine*. Durham, NC: Duke University Press.

Becker, G. 1997. *Disrupted Lives: How People Create Meaning in a Chaotic World*. Berkeley: University of California Press.

Bloch, M. and J. Parry. 1989. 'Introduction: Money and the Morality of Exchange', in P. Parry and M. Bloch (eds), *Money and the Morality of Exchange*. Cambridge: Cambridge University Press.

Bury, M. 1982. 'Chronic Illness as Biographical Disruption', *Sociology of Health and Illness* 4(2): 167–82.

Capra, F. 2002. *The Hidden Connections*. London: Harper Collins.

______. 2005. 'Complexity and Life', *Theory, Culture and Society* 22: 33–44.

Cilliers, P. 1988. *Complexity and Postmodernism: Understanding Complex Systems*. London: Routledge.

______. 2005. 'Complexity, Deconstruction and Relativism', *Theory, Culture and Society* 22: 255–67.

Diamond, J. 2005. *Collapse: How Societies Choose to Fail or Succeed*. London: Penguin.

Douglas, M. 1975. *Implicit Meanings: Essays in Anthropology*. London: Routledge.

______. 1992. *Risk and Blame: Essays in Cultural Theory*. London: Routledge.

Gupta, A. and J. Ferguson (eds). 1997. *Anthropological Locations: Boundaries and Grounds of a Field Science*. Berkeley: University of California Press.

Habermas, J. 1971. *Knowledge and Human Interests*. Boston, MA: Beacon Press.

Hamilton, M. 2001. *The Sociology of Religion: Theoretical and Comparative Perspectives*. London: Routledge.

Hand, W.D. 1980. *Magical Medicine*. Berkeley: University of California Press.

Harding Clark Report. 2006. 'The Lourdes Hospital Inquiry: An Inquiry into Peripartum Hysterectomy at Our Lady of Lourdes Hospital, Drogheda', report of Judge Maureen Harding Clark Sc. Dublin: Stationery Office.

Held, D., A. McGrew. D. Goldblatt and J. Perraton. 1999. *Global Transformations: Politics, Economics and Culture*. Cambridge: Polity.

House of Lords. 2000. 'Complementary and Alternative Medicine', report of the Select Committee on Science and Technology, HL Paper 123. London: HMSO.

Illich, I. 1976. *Limits to Medicine. Medical Nemesis: The Expropriation of Health*. Harmondsworth: Penguin.

Kleinman, A. 1980. *Patients and Healers in the Context of Culture*. Berkeley: University of California Press.

Luhmann, N. 1993. *Risk: A Sociological Theory*. Berlin: De Gruyter.

McClean, S. 2003. 'Doctoring the Spirit: Exploring the Use and Meaning of Mimicry and Parody at a Healing Centre in the North Of England', *Health* 7(4): 483–500.

McQuaide, M. 2005. 'The Rise of Alternative Health Care: A Sociological Account', *Social Theory and Health* 3(4): 286–301.

Mathews, H.F. 1987. 'Rootwork: Description of an Ethnomedical System of the American South', *Southern Medical Journal* 80: 885–91.

Maurer, B. 2006. 'The Anthropology of Money', *Annual Review of Anthropology* 35: 15-36.

Melitz, J. 1970. 'The Polanyi School of Anthropology of Money: an Economist's View', *American Anthropologist* 72(5): 1020–1040.

Navarro, V. 1986. *Crisis, Health and Medicine*. London: Tavistock.

Peters, D., H. Andrews and D. Hills. 2006. 'Integrating Complementary Medicine into Primary Care: An Audit of Five Months' Referrals to the Get Well U.K. Complimentary Therapy Service in South Islington', London: unpublished report.

Rapport, N. and A. Dawson (eds). 1998. *Migrants of Identity: Perceptions of Home in a World of Movement*. Oxford: Berg.

Robinson, N. 2006. 'Get Well U.K.: Does it Work? A Pilot Project Investigating the Integration of Complementary Medicine into Primary Care',. London: unpublished independent auditor's report

Shapiro, F. 2001. *Eye Movement Desensitization and Reprocessing: Basic Principles, Protocols and Procedures*. New York: Guilford Press.

Shapiro, F. and M. Forrest. 2004. *EMDR: The Break-through 'Eye Movement' Therapy for Overcoming Anxiety Stress and Trauma*. New York: Basic Books.

Searle, J. 1996. *The Construction of Social Reality*. London: Penguin.

Sharma, U. 1995. *Complementary Medicine Today: Practitioners and Patients*. London: Routledge.

Simmel, G. 1990 [1907]. *Philosophy of Money*. London: Routledge.

Sullivan, D. 2001. *Cosmetic Surgery: The Cutting Edge of Medicine in America*. New Brunswick, NJ: Rutgers University Press.

Szasz, T. 1961. *The Myth of Mental Illness: Foundations of a Theory of Personal Conduct*. London: Secker.

Sztompka, P. 1999. *Trust: A Sociological Theory*. Cambridge: Cambridge University Press.

Thomas, K. 1973. *Religion and the Decline of Magic*. London: Penguin.

Trevor-Roper, H. 2006. *Europe's Physician: The Various Life of Sir Theodore De Mayerne*. New Haven, CT: Yale University Press.

Vaskilampi, T. 1981. 'Culture and Folk Medicine', in T. Vaskilampi and C. MacCormack (eds), *Folk Medicine and Health Culture: The Role of Folk Medicine in Modern Health Care*. Kuopio: Department of Community Health, University of Kuopio.

Vattimo, G. 1991. *The End of Modernity: Nihilism and Hermeneutics in Post-modern Culture*. Cambridge: Polity Press.

WHO. 2002. 'WHO Traditional Medicine Strategy, 2002–2005'. Geneva: World Health Organization.

Zabala, S. (ed.) 2006. *Weakening Philosophy: Essays in Honour of Gianni Vattimo*. Montreal: McGill-Queen's University Press.

Notes on Contributors

Editors

Dr Ronnie Moore.

Ronnie Moore comes from Belfast. He has lived in the South of Germany and Australia and was Senior lecturer at St Bartholomew and the Royal London Hospitals, University of London before returning to Ireland. He currently lectures in Medical Anthropology and Sociology in the Schools of Public Health Medicine and Population Science and Sociology at University College Dublin.

Dr Stuart McClean.

Stuart McClean is a Senior Lecturer based in the Department of Health, Community and Policy Studies at UWE, Bristol. His book, *An Ethnography of Crystal and Spiritual Healers in Northern England: marginal medicine and mainstream concerns*, is published by Edwin Mellen Press.

Contributors

The book is informed by experts from a variety of academic disciplines. Dr Catherine Cox is a medical historian and is based in the Centre for the History of Medicine in Ireland, School of History and Archives, at UCD, Dublin. Dr Sue Philpin is Senior Lecturer, Head of Centre for Primary Care, Public Health and Older People, at Swansea University. Dr Anne Macfarlane is Lecturer in Primary Care, at the National University of Ireland, Galway. Dr Tomas de Brún is an anthropologist and researcher based at the National University of Ireland. Dr Ayo Wahlberg is based at the new centre for the study of bioscience, biomedicine, biotechnology and society – the London School of Economics. Dr Geraldine Lee-Treweek is a

Principal Lecturer in Applied Social Studies in the Department of Interdisciplinary Studies, Manchester Metropolitan University. Professor Julie Stone is Deputy Director of the Council for Healthcare Regulatory Excellence. Julie is a barrister and medical ethicist and has contributed to numerous initiatives in health policy and law, held Secretary of State appointments, and published extensively in her field. Her books include: *Complementary Medicine and the Law*, (1996) Oxford University Press (with Joan Mathews), *An Ethical Framework for Complementary and Alternative Therapists*, (2002) Routledge, and *Psychotherapy and the Law*, Whurr (2004) (with Peter Jenkins and Vincent Keter).

Index